Chris Lynch &
Michelle Tackabery

Within Your
REACH

A Journey through Diabetes

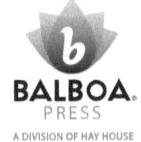

BALBOA
PRESS

A DIVISION OF HAY HOUSE

ISBN: 978-1-4525-6444-9 (sc)
ISBN: 978-1-4525-6445-6 (e)

Balboa Press books may be ordered through booksellers or by contacting:

Balboa Press
A Division of Hay House
1663 Liberty Drive
Bloomington, IN 47403
www.balboapress.com
1-(877) 407-4847

Because of the dynamic nature of the Internet, any web addresses or links contained in this book may have changed since publication and may no longer be valid. The views expressed in this work are solely those of the author and do not necessarily reflect the views of the publisher, and the publisher hereby disclaims any responsibility for them.

The author of this book does not dispense medical advice or prescribe the use of any technique as a form of treatment for physical, emotional, or medical problems without the advice of a physician, either directly or indirectly. The intent of the author is only to offer information of a general nature to help you in your quest for emotional and spiritual well-being. In the event you use any of the information in this book for yourself, which is your constitutional right, the author and the publisher assume no responsibility for your actions.

Some of the names in this book have been changed.

Printed in the United States of America

Balboa Press rev. date: 12/19/2012

PREFACE

The first step is the hardest.

When I was 16 years old, I went camping one spring weekend with my boyfriend in the Blue Ridge Mountains of North Carolina. We were with a large group of trusted friends in an area near Blowing Rock, named for the never-ceasing winds that buffet the peaks. We hiked for about an hour up a narrow, rocky path until we came upon a clearing with several ledges. The ledges stood between 80 and 150 feet above the next landfall, and were popular with rock climbers who did what we were going to do: learn rappelling. Well, my boyfriend was going to learn. I had no intention of jumping off a perfectly good mountain; I was scared of the fall. My boyfriend was absolutely terrified, which was why he was going to do it. He hated heights. He got nauseous close to the top of down escalators and couldn't bear to stand near balcony railings. But he wanted to conquer his fear. So he was going to wear a bicycle helmet, strap himself up in what looked to me like a terribly complicated and extremely thin harness made of acrylic, buckle himself in with a couple of carabiners to a thick rope tied to an ancient tree, and step off a mountain nearly 5,000 feet above sea level. At the campsite that morning, he had looked at me and croaked weakly, "We who are about to die . . ." I didn't laugh. The hike had seen my mouth dry up like an abandoned creek and my stomach roil with acidic worry. Images of him slipping, falling, reaching out to me, and closing his eyes forever would not escape my mind.

Well. I was sixteen.

Three members of our group helped him get attached to the rope, speaking to each other in that guy talk that fails to comfort bystanders— "Don't worry, if you die I won't drive your car, I'll sell it instead; dibs on your girlfriend; if you start to fall, fall on your face, you'll look better;" that kind of stuff. I couldn't watch. I went to the edge of a small ledge away from them and looked down at the ground.

A rustle of fabric and the clink of metal interrupted my torturous thoughts, and I looked over to see my too-thin boyfriend standing up on the ledge, facing away from the sky, and breathing out loudly through his mouth. I called his name, but he didn't look at me. One of the guys going down with him, a "babysitter," suddenly jumped backwards off the ledge. I gasped.

"I'll be down here, 'bout ten feet off your five o'clock," he hollered.

To my boyfriend's right was his boss, a man who was his second father, his best friend, his – well, you can figure it out, I guess. He looked over at me, "Don't worry, we got him," he said in a low voice.

"I know," I answered. But I didn't. I was afraid.

He looked at my boyfriend. "The first step is the hardest," the older man said. "Which foot first?"

"Left," he said.

"Left," the older man repeated.

My boyfriend picked up his left foot, and took one step back. His foot landed about a foot behind and below him, somewhere beyond the ledge. With one more step, the lower half of his body disappeared below the ledge. I heard a sound I couldn't recognize — a groan, maybe. I could still see his face, but it was turned toward the older man.

"I've known you all my life," the older man said. "And I know how to tie a rope and harness."

He nodded. Then he jumped backwards, and disappeared.

I ran to a vantage point on another ledge. He was halfway down the mountain's edge in a crouch, both feet against the stone. He was smiling, because he knew that his rope and harness were secure, and his friends would catch him if he fell. In a few steps, he had journeyed from fear to faith.

I've known Chris Lynch since that same time in my life. Back then, he never seemed afraid of anything, or worried, or upset. Things seemed to roll off him like the proverbial water off a duck. He smiled all the time. He laughed and joked.

Same as now, really. Except . . .

Back then, Chris was playing a series of parts: the good son, the best friend, the obedient Catholic. The kindest, most content human being alive. But inside, he was afraid. He didn't believe that he could ever step off his own ledge into the unknown. He grew to have music, family, friends who loved him. The decent, All-American life we're all supposed to want —a fantastic, high-paying job with a prestigious firm, a pretty fiancée, a showcase house. But every single day—every single breath—he was waiting for a shadow to fall across his life. A shadow he thought was going to wreck everything. When that shadow did, finally, fall, he discovered that his fear had already done the wrecking for him.

Chris didn't need to learn how to conquer fear. He had to embrace it, walk with it and listen to it. And when he did, he realized something amazing. Not a secret. Not a key to life, the universe, and everything. Just the simplest things, the thing that children have and lose: faith, and joy.

Joy is on the other side of this journey you are about to take with us, but have confidence. We know how to tie a rope and harness.

Michelle Tackabery
Sunday, November 18, 2012

1

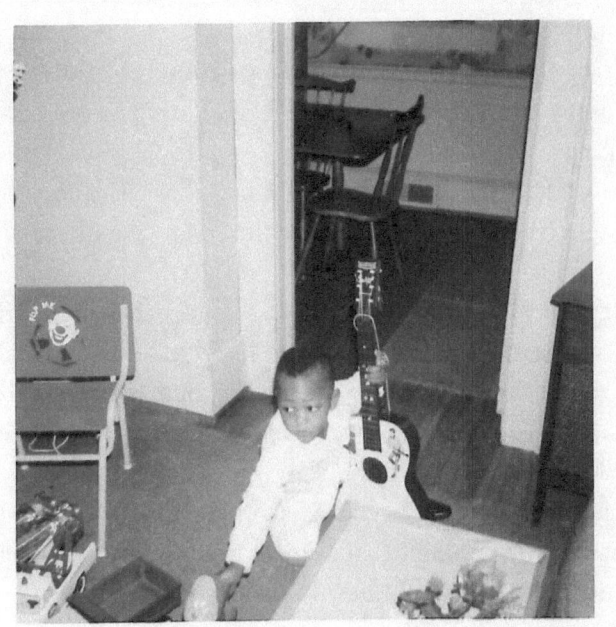

ONSET

The onset happened Sunday and
Monday; really bad on Monday.

This is not just another story about diabetes.

I felt like death. Which was indescribably bad. I had decided it was probably the flu. I was feverish and could not stop drinking. I could not get enough liquid in me. I just Was. Not. Right.

My cousin Tony and I had gone to lunch, and I remember drinking six, maybe seven glasses of pink lemonade, but it still wasn't enough. Tony had this weird look on his face, as if he wanted to say, "Chris, you don't look right." But I wasn't in the mood to receive that, so we just didn't deal with it. We went to see the movie *W.*, and I remember that I kept getting up and going to the bathroom.

Now, in the back of my mind, I was thinking, "Diabetes!" In the forefront of my mind, I was thinking, "Nah, I just have the flu." I couldn't stop drinking.

When we left the movie, Tony still had that weird look on his face, and I thought, this is the beginning of the end.

I went home, by myself, to my big ass house. The nearest friend to me was Tom, who lived eight houses down. I said to him, "Dude, I'm feeling thirsty; I've got the flu, can you go get me some stuff?" So Tom kindly brought me a two-liter bottle of orange soda, or maybe it was lemonade; I loved any kind of sugary drink.

I felt feverish and flu-ish, but what I was actually feeling was death. My organs were beginning to shut down, but I didn't know that. By early Tuesday morning, though, I knew I was in real trouble.

About two o'clock in the morning, I felt so utterly awful and alone. I was so listless and lethargic, it took every ounce of energy to get to the master bathroom, turn the water on and sit my body in the Jacuzzi. My body was so cold that I thought if I sat in the hot water, it would make me feel better. My thirst was so overpowering that instead I turned on the faucet of cold water, and drank, and drank, and drank. Still, no matter how much water I swallowed, I could not quench my thirst. I'm not sure how long it took me to even try to get out of the tub, my body was so listless and unresponsive. Eventually, I did get out after several attempts. I was strangely calm, even though my heart seemed out of rhythm in my body. I remember that I said, "Okay Lord, I'm going to sleep. Good night and God bless." I didn't say goodbye, but I just went to sleep. In my mind, I had the flu, and the flu is one of those things that can't be helped by a visit to the hospital or the doctor.

Now, every day Momma Cille and I had an eight o'clock call. All the grandkids had their time to call our grandmother, whom we called Momma Cille, or Ma, and mine was eight o'clock a.m. When I didn't call at eight o'clock, Momma Cille assumed the worst. I had missed the call by about 45 minutes. When it came to me and the other grandkids, she had that motherly instinct.

Ma called me, but I wasn't able to answer my phone. She was worried, so she sent Blanche out to the house. Blanche Jackson was Ma's nurse who had cared for Ma's daughter, my Aunt Phyllis; when Aunt Phyllis passed, Blanche stayed on with Momma Cille, and had become her caretaker, confidante and a best friend; she was devoted to Ma, getting Ma's walker for her and helping get around.

Ma said to Blanche, "Get out to Chris's house; just get out there. He is not doing well; I need to get him to that doctor." My doctor's name was Dr. Richard Dougherty, pronounced "dock-er-tee," but Ma always pronounced it "dock-er-ee." She couldn't say it correctly, so she couldn't spell it to find his number, either. Ma called Mary Richardson, a dear friend of the family, who helped her to look up my doctor's name, and then Blanche drove out to my house, picked me up and took me to the doctor's office.

I was pretty calm, trying to make jokes like I always do—I was still me, but it took every ounce of energy I had to put my pants on. Blanche was keeping it together, but even Blanche had a scared look on her face when she saw me moving so slowly, like, "Oh, shit!" I didn't know I looked puffy, extraordinarily ill and weak. People usually don't see me like that. They see me up; the leader, outgoing, that kind of stuff. But I was, frankly, fucked up.

I was afraid to call 911, or a hospital, or anyone I knew. I didn't have health insurance, and I didn't have much money, so I said to myself, "Well, I guess this is the way I'm supposed to go. Lord, I trust you. If you want me to stay around, then You'll take care of it in the way that You always take care of everything." And I let the worry go.

Mary, a nurse at the doctor's office, took one look at me and instantly knew what was happening. When you have diabetic ketoacidosis, you have a fruity smell to your breath from the citrus coming out of the acidity in the body. She said, "Chris, you need to go to the hospital. I'm calling them right now to get a trauma room ready for you."

I said okay, and then she said, "Can you walk?" I said yes, and that's about the last bit of energy that I exerted that day.

I was going deeper into a kind of fog. My body was falling apart. I think they say your brain is the last thing to go, but the way I was breathing, it was as if I was about to go into cardiac arrest. It had a heavy, yet shallow, rhythm. Blanche was scared, and as she got more frightened, she started driving faster. I remember that when we pulled into the emergency room entrance, I heard the tires screech! My brother Damion and I always used to make jokes about Batman when we were kids, and how the Batmobile would always make that sound. I thought, "This must be really bad if Blanche has to drive like the Batman!"

When I got into the emergency room, I thought, "God, You know I don't have health insurance. I'm totally in Your hands." One of the nurses in the ER asked, "How do you feel Mr. Lynch?" I responded with something of an understatement: "I've been feeling bad since Thursday," and collapsed on the gurney. *"Feeling bad since Thursday"* was written in my medical records and listed as my chief complaint: But it was much worse than that.

I was almost dead when I got to the hospital. My body was depleted of insulin, so it had no fuel to drawn on. My body was breaking down the fats for energy instead, which caused acids known as ketones to build up in my blood and urine until they reached poisonous levels My blood had become acidic to the point that it was killing me.

A "normal" fasting blood glucose level, which just means a level reading taken before you eat, is less than 100 milligrams per deciliter (mg/dl), and one hour after eating a meal, a normal level is less than 140 mg/dl in most people. Glucose is a carbohydrate that provides instant energy to the body, and is found in table sugar and other foods. The standard glucose tolerance test, or GTT, can return a diagnosis of diabetes if your blood glucose level is greater than or equal to 200 mg/dl two hours after ingesting glucose, but usually patients have to be tested more than once to be sure.[1]

---

1 Alan L. Rubin, MD, *Diabetes for Dummies, 2nd Edition*, Wiley Publishing, 2004.

Later, my doctors would tell me that my blood sugar must have been over 300 mg/dl for at least the past few months, which meant that I had been coasting on the edge of death for more than three months. The crisis grew worse, and worse, and finally my body was at a breaking point.

I remember clearly, though, what happened next. I'd said a prayer, right before I'd fallen on the gurney. I prayed, "God, if this is my time to go, thank You for everything You've done in my life. I believe in your son, Jesus. Forgive me of my sins, and welcome me into Your kingdom."

As soon as I released this prayer, I felt an overwhelming warmth and peace. Even though I was in pain, my body aching, my spirit was untouched. There was no out of body experience, but I felt strangely calm, to the point that it must have been irritating to those who were helping me. In this moment bridging the now and the hereafter, life seemed suspended, there was nothing else to be, to strive for and the ego no longer existed. I felt the end of pride. I am lying totally naked, everybody's pulling and poking and tucking and sticking and pricking—I could fight it, or "let go and let God." Once I said that prayer, I don't think I passed out or went unconscious, I was at peace and at the place where I could release and say, "Okay. I'm in Your care now. I'm in God's hands and whoever, whatever my fate and destiny is, I accept it."

I was grateful for the gurney, because I felt that finally I could rest. So I collapsed and allowed myself to be vulnerable. As an ER nurse opened the IV units she said to me, "Mr. Lynch, you have severe diabetic ketoacidosis." She added, "You have no more blood. Your blood is acid."

My mind went down a strange path when she used the term "acid." I thought about my favorite fruit: oranges. When I'd heard about the reference to citrus, I thought, "I like lemons and limes and oranges, and my blood is basically lemons and limes and oranges—acid!" Next, my mind threw music into the mix; I thought about acid rock, then I progressed to acid rain, and finally back to citrus. I also thought, "I have citrusy breath!" Randomly I thought about one of my favorites, lemon-lime orange pound cake and how good it sounded right about now. That led me to a Paula Deen episode where she made orange brownies. My mind was a video stream of fruity desserts, fruit and citrus. Clearly I had no idea about the magnitude of what was happening to me But then I thought with alarm, "Wait, I have no blood?" At this point, they deeply infused me with multiple bags of insulin. Although I didn't have to get a blood transfusion, since I hadn't lost any blood, they were working hard to reactivate my blood.

I was truly in the beginning stages of cardiac arrest; that's why I had that panting, scary breathing. They gave me oxygen; I felt the ER tube loops being placed into my nose. I remember feeling cold but also the sensation of warmth. The nurse informed me that my organs were in the process of shutting down. I now know that when your organs begin to shut down, your body begins to fade. Like a dead person, your body starts cooling, and my temperature had dropped to 92 degrees Fahrenheit. The warmth was coming from a hypothermia blanket that had been placed over me. I was conscious, but I was going in and out. I heard someone saying, "He's not doing too well, get down here!" That's when Dr. Arfana A. Kishan came in. When she got there, she was looking at the chart, then looking at me, then looking at the chart. My eyes popped open, and I said, "Hey Doc!"

She jumped as if I had just scared her to death, and said, "Mr. Lynch, I thought you were dying!"

I asked, "Is this heaven?" She laughed. The comedian in me was still there. "How am I doing? Am I going to make it? Am I moving in the right direction?" I asked. She said, "Yes, but you still have a long way to go."

And then she said the word *diabetes*.

Let's just say when I finally go to a hospital, y'all, I make damned sure it's a life-and-death, bona fide emergency.

About six months before, I had left a well-paying, secure job at a Charlotte, North Carolina bank—and all the stress of the corporate bullshit that came with it—to start my own electronics consulting business. I was on fire with creativity, which seemed to be flowing constantly. Ideas, money-making ideas, just seemed to come from everywhere.

My typical day began at eight in the morning and ended at two o'clock at night. Music or the TV was on all the time. I was always on the phone, always searching the Internet and always some kind of background noise for added stimulation. Suddenly I would look at my watch and notice, "Oh shit, I haven't eaten."

My body was starving for food, and what did I typically do? I took whatever was most convenient to stop the hunger and went to get it as fast as I could with no thought about calories, diet, sodium intake or nutritional value. My life had a rhythm of food, eat, work; food, eat, work. And, I must admit that after separating with the woman I had once asked to be my second wife, in the absence of sex, this busy life was all that I had left. When you don't have sex as an outlet, it's easy to tell yourself on some level, "Well, I can replace it with something else." As a result, I often ended up working this way at least six days a week, never really taking a day off.

Momma Cille would say as she took my hand in hers, "Now Chris, I notice you're getting puffy and you're gaining weight." Other people would also comment, "You're gaining weight, Chris." Inside I was a bit panicky and thinking, "Oh, shit!" But I'd brush it off to deal with it later. I'd say something like, "Yeah, I should start walking." My cousin Tony kept talking about exercise and ways to get healthier, but I kept telling him, "Tony, I'm busy. Once I get this thing kicked off, I'll do it." It was my point of determination to get my business launched. But that little voice inside suspected the worst. "I'm out of control. I'm spiraling out of control."

I didn't feel good about how I was living, but I felt that I needed to be on my own. People had always said, throughout my career, that "Chris has an incredible work ethic, because he works his ass off. But I knew my blood pressure was high. Financial woes would hit, and hit, and hit, and it felt to me like my body was an air pump, just imploding and blowing up stress and more stress.

Now I never felt like I was going to have a heart attack, but I felt puffy, and salty, and out of control—strained, stressed and worn out. But I never really connected the dots on how to get in control, and part of it felt good, because I knew that something would eventually come to help bring me back. I didn't realize it was going to be intensive care. I thought I was going to need to go back to therapy, sit down with a therapist, open up, talk about things, call it a day and move on with my life. But nope! That was not the case.

Dr. Kishan told me, "Mr. Lynch, we can't figure out if you have Type 1 or Type 2 diabetes."

I had walked into Carolinas Medical Center-Pineville (CMC-Pineville) at 11:00 a.m. on Tuesday, October 21, 2008, but the medical staff had been unsuccessful at getting an accurate blood glucose level reading until just after 12 p.m. When they got the reading, they were knocked out. They told me they thought it was the highest reading in medical history.

Dr. Kishan said to me that in medical school, the highest blood glucose level she had ever seen was about 684 milligrams per decaliter (mg/dl). She said that person had died. I had to face the fear that I had pushed away my entire life, a fear born in my childhood when my brother Damion and I would get our bath, and my grandfather would have to check the sugar in his urine. I remembered seeing him with his Bayer branded urine sticks, and always being afraid of having to check my own urine someday, and stick myself with needles to give myself insulin like he did. I didn't want to know what my sugar was. But she told me anyway.

My blood glucose level was 1469 mg/dl.

2

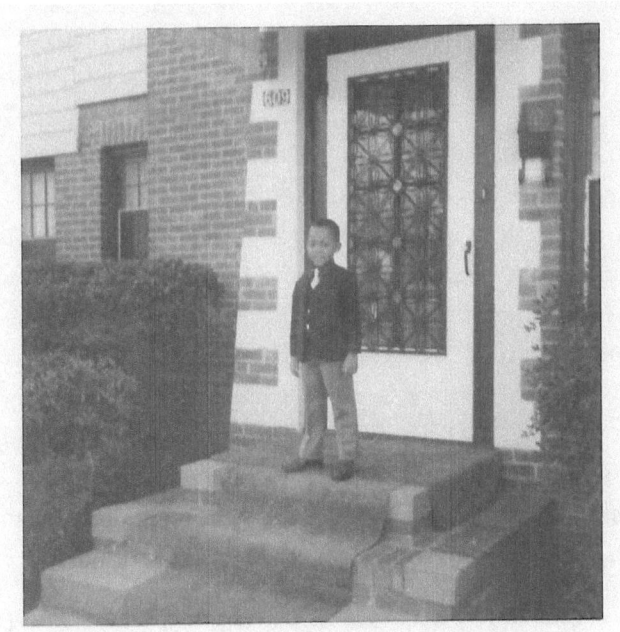

609

---

609 Baldwin Avenue in Charlotte, where
we grew up, is the headquarters.

My brother Damion and I always refer to it as 609. The earliest memory
that I can recall is when I was maybe three years old; I was born in 1966,
so that earliest memory is in 1969. I was in the basement of 609, Ma's
house, and I was dribbling a basketball. I remember my Uncle Art—Art
Jr., Ma's youngest son and my mother's brother—and his good friend

Chuck were there. I could smell either incense or pot, or both of them, together. I think the incense was what I smelled mostly, but I am pretty sure pot was involved!

One of three songs was playing; I don't remember which one, but when I think about it, I remember the bands War and Three Dog Night. It was either "Why Can't We Be Friends," by War, or "Shambala," or "Joy to the World" by Three Dog Night. I remember dribbling a basketball, smelling incense, smiling, and being happy. That is my earliest memory. To this day, I've always had a fondness for that late 60s, early 70s music, especially like Three Dog Night and War and those kind of bands.

Music and faith to me are not synonymous, but I'll tell you—I really believe music is the peanut butter layer of life. Music is God's reminder, to me, of Him on earth, and it comes in so many expressions—kind of like He does. From 20th century rock bands like The Police, to Dieterich Buxtehude, a 15th century German composer the equivalent of Keith Emerson or Gregg Allman, who wrote this incredible music I often hear during mass at the Basilica of the Immaculate Conception in Washington, D.C. Classical organ music moves me as much as hearing my favorite group Van Halen's "Unchained," or "Jump." Every kind and everything about music speaks to me, moves my soul.

My Mom Patricia had a brain aneurysm and died ten days after I was born, so I never knew her. What I know of her is through stories from other people. You know when people ask you, "If you had one thing in life to wish for that you don't have now, what would it be?" If there's one thing in life that I wish I could have, it would be the chance to meet my Mom.

But I got a lot of her through Momma Cille and my grandfather Arthur. Damion and I were told that, as my Mom had her aneurysm, her dying words, which she told the nursing supervisor at the hospital in NC where I was born, were, "Tell my Mom to raise my boys, and teach 'em their prayers." My grandmother and grandfather were in Chicago visiting relatives when they heard about what happened, and they just hightailed it back to North Carolina to take care of us.

"No cross, no crown" was Momma Cille's mantra. Ma was a deeply spiritual person, so in her mind the struggle of Jesus on the Cross, the struggle of the Passion, and all of that, leads you to the crown of Victory.

Momma Cille told me many times that her goal in life was to follow what her daughter asked her to do for Damion and me. That's why the prayer that I will always remember was the one she taught us. It was the Guardian Angel prayer.

Angel of God, my guardian dear,
to whom God's love commits me here,
ever this day be at my side,
To watch, to lead, to guard, to guide.

I still say this prayer every day.

The only death that I would experience directly when I was a child was the death of Momma Cille's mother, Odessa. We had a family reunion recently, and looking through some photos, and I found one of me from that time. My face showed a bubbly, bouncing, happy kid somewhat oblivious in the midst of all that sorrow.

As a result of all that happened, Momma Cille was over-protective of me and Damion. Damion and I both felt we weren't allowed to have fun. Sometimes I mourn the fact that I wasn't allowed to be a kid, to be free, to even fall and scrape my knee. Don't get me wrong—I had a great childhood in many respects and I feel very blessed—but the fact is, I didn't have a whole lot of fun the way most kids did at that age.

St. Patrick's Cathedral in Charlotte, North Carolina, was where our family went to church. My Mom, her sister Phyllis, and brother Art Jr. were known as the first black kids to integrate Roman Catholic schools in Charlotte. They went to O'Donoghue School, before it was renamed St. Patrick's School, and Damion and I went when it became St. Pat's. My cousins, Patrick and Deirdre, went too.

I started kindergarten at St. Pat's and attended through the eighth grade, and St. Pat's is one of the two places on this earth where I feel the strongest connections, faith-wise; the other is the Basilica in Washington, D.C. I have an overwhelming, crystal-clear channel to God in those places. I am not distracted at all by other troubles; I can go there and just feel the presence.

You don't miss mass; that was our family creed. If you are dying, you find a way to get the Eucharist. Even when we traveled, we went to mass. We *never* missed mass. Our itinerary would be to find the hotel, and then find the closest Catholic Church to it. Momma Cille, if she ever granted any kind of preferential treatment to anybody, it was because they were Catholic. All of her kids would go to Catholic school. She knew all the priests; all the bishops.

We were all active in the church—youth ministry, music ministry; I mean everything. Faith for us was prayer; we always prayed. For example, I always get down on my knees before the stroke of midnight on New Year's Eve and say a prayer for the coming year, and that was something my grandfather instilled in us that I still do. My grandfather was my confirmation sponsor. Everything tied into faith and the church. Everything did.

Momma Cille always made sure that Damion and I stayed busy and involved in extracurricular activities. Not activities where we might get hurt, like sports, but art and music. Damion and I were always taught together. Ma never wanted us to be competitive against each other, so if I took piano, Damion took piano. One year Damion and I were given a Wurlitzer organ as a Christmas present, and it sits at 609 to this day. It has been there for 30-plus years. We learned organ and piano for three or four years, but I eventually got bored with it.

There's a picture of me somewhere when we were given little toy guitars for Christmas one year, and I was doing a kind of Pete Townshend impression with mine. I didn't even know who Pete Townshend was at the time, but I just connected with the guitar in that kind of way. So there's this picture of me in this little robe, and I have this little guitar and I'm doing this move like I'm going to destroy it. Damion calls it my Pete Townshend picture.

At the time, I didn't realize that I was making a metaphysical connection to that instrument. But I'd always had an ear for music; I can hear a tone and I know which chord it is. My brother Damion is much more of an accomplished musician than I am. He is the one who can read music, and he sings professionally in the Washington Chorus. But when it comes to notes and chords, I can hear a piece of music and I will know that one sound is an A; one's A-Flat, one's G, one's G-Flat, one's F, one's F-Sharp. I guess I've been bitten by the bug.

During my piano lessons, I could never read the music I was supposed to learn, but I could memorize things quickly. Our music teacher, Charlie Friar, was a very famous keyboardist in Charlotte, and he was the first person that got me excited about playing music. Charlie gave Damion and me private lessons down the street from St. Pat's.

Around fifth or sixth grade there was a lady at St. Pat's, Cathy Topping who was the guitar teacher, and I thought she was really amazing. She was blonde, she had these wire-rimmed glasses, and she played acoustic and classical guitar, and all of her students idolized her. We thought she was the coolest, and she taught us the popular folk songs of the late '70s played at mass.

When the group that played music at 5:30 mass on Saturday nights stopped, Damion and I were part of the group that was asked to become what affectionately became known as the St. Patrick's Folk Group. To this day, people still remember us, and I am blown away because God truly used us as instruments. When I first saw twanging on guitars at mass, I was into it, always asking questions, like, "How do you play that chord again?"

Miss Topping taught us the songs that to this day I still love, all the old Catholic songs, and the songs we mastered evolved as we moved on further. After Cathy Topping, Jeff Hildreth and Eddie Norris, who were in the old folk group, hung out with us, and they became our idols for music. Jeff was the one that taught me about the electric guitar. My influences then were B.B. King, Chuck Berry and Johnny Cash. Those guys just blew me away.

Johnny Cash taught me how to strum. I remember Johnny Paycheck, who wrote, "Take This Job and Shove it." Those simple songs they played just resonated with me. Soon everything we did around music evolved in church. That was where our talent came out, and we were the ones that could really take the new music, the "Glory and Praise" music that was part of the mass in the Diocese of Charlotte then, and mess with it. We could improvise with it, and make it cool. Jeff and Eddie gave us permission to be cool at mass; to add a little bit here and there, you know.

We took one "Holy, Holy (Sanctus)[2]" that was called the "Missa Bossa Nova[3]," and we messed with it and called our version the "Missalette Jam." The songs we played were like the greatest hits in our missalettes, and we memorized them all. They were all guitar-driven. The "Glory and Praise" music gave us a foundation into the harder stuff we wanted to learn how to play; they became like our Led Zeppelin, and the Who. Our influences would always be in our mass music, somewhere, someway, somehow.

I believe that when you open yourself up to the mystery and the reality of God, it is shown to you. Some people absorb it from the trees, some people from books; I get it from music and sound and from high mass. Those are my reminders of what the Mystery is.

Damion and I were always referred to as the Blues Brothers, because we both played from the same amp. Damion was always simple where I was always richer, more complex with sound. What I mean by "complex" with sound was that I had four or five gadgets in my rig. Damion would just have a cord from his bass right into the amp and would turn it up; that's how he played. So his stuff never broke! Damion's rig was very simple. I was the one who had to have racks and pedals and all kinds of gadgets.

Damion always said I had a very distinct sound in my guitar-playing, and my good friend and band mate Mike, who is a drummer, said the same thing. You know how they say Eric Clapton and Eddie Van Halen have their "sound?" I have a very distinct sound that identifies me. To this day, I kind of know what it is, but I let others talk about what it is, because I'm just doing it, being it. It's hard for me to define it.

For most of my life, all of my decisions—all of my day-to-day things—were overshadowed by fear. If Ma said come in and do something, I did it without question even if it caused me some kind of pain, like not playing ball with the other kids even if they made fun of me for sitting out. I think I began to equate pain and happiness in a synonymous way, because Ma said I had to experience pain, as Jesus did on the Cross, to get the crown of heaven.

---

2 Part of the Roman Catholic Eucharistic Prayer, "Holy, Holy (Sanctus)" can be spoken or sung by the congregation. The complete text is "Holy, holy, holy Lord, God of power and might, Heaven and earth are full of your glory. Hosanna in the highest. Blessed is he who comes in the name of the Lord. Hosanna in the highest."

3 "Missa Bossa Nova" was composed by Rev. Peter Schotles and recorded in 1968.

At this stage, I didn't realize that I didn't have a mother because Momma Cille was my mother in every way. My family spoke about a lady named Patricia, who was my mother, but I didn't put everything together about who she was to me until later in life.

The discipline in my family came from my Aunt Phyllis first, and then Momma Cille. Aunt Phyllis lived at 609 with Momma Cille, my grandfather Arthur, Momma Cille's sister Alma, Damion, and I. Art Jr. was there for a time, but he did the Greg Brady thing. He lived in his own room, apart from us, and then left when he had "grown up" and found his own place. Except his room wasn't in the attic; it was in the basement. We were two young boys and we often got spankings and punishments, but most of my fear was 60 percent of Aunt Phyllis, and 40 percent of Momma Cille.

With Aunt Phyllis, I experienced the pure fear of being punished for anything I might do wrong, because she always expected me to be a serious little gentleman. At the same time, she was the one that would nurture me by buying me the things that I would need to grow as a person—clothes, school supplies, musical instruments. Aunt Phyllis was very active in the civil rights movement and the Democratic Party in Charlotte. I admired Aunt Phyllis, but there was a time when she was also the one that I was afraid of the most.

One of my most scarring events was when Aunt Phyllis took away my stereo. I don't remember what I did to deserve the punishment; I don't even remember how old I was. I was a kid, so I'd talk back occasionally, of course, but I never did drugs, I never smoked, and I never ran away. When I'd watch television shows back then, some kid would always be running away from home, but I never did that.

Music is life for me, and that day she took it away for a year. I was so fearful of her not letting me have my music back at the end of the year that even when I was by myself in the car, I didn't turn on the radio. As I was getting older and hanging around my friends at church and school more, playing at mass, and doing things in the world outside of 609's environment, I would sometimes stop and think, "Wow, what am I so afraid of?"

To survive, emotionally, I just did what Aunt Phyllis told me to do, which was to suppress my childish excitement and joy. I learned to be the opposite, a process that left me enamored by fear, if that's even possible to say. I worried constantly about doing the wrong thing. In the absence of music

I became very creative in my mind, in my heart, and in my prayer life—my spirit life. So in a strange way, the punishment became a blessing. I didn't know that's what I was doing, but I always felt a connection to God, so I always had some kind of communication going on with Him. Music was my life. The day she gave it back to me, I felt like I could breathe again.

Ma said to me once, "Chris, I don't want you going to the baseball field up the street, because you might become like the kids that are around you." Ma and Aunt Phyllis were so over-protective of my brother and me that when we would go on Boy Scout trips, Aunt Phyllis would pay what I used to call her crew—people who worked with her in her non-profit group—to go with us to make sure Damion and I were okay. Other kids called us The Princes. The Princes, or the Blues Brothers, that's what they called us. Being chaperoned was just Momma Cille's and Phyllis' way to fulfill my Mom's instruction: teach my boys their prayers and raise 'em. So that's what they did, to the best of their knowledge.

Now some of that sucked, because when I'm sitting next to one of the other guys, I'm thinking, "Well, shit, if you don't have a chaperone, why do I?" You know, I had an eight o'clock curfew on a date one time. That isn't normal! What kind of girl wants to date you when you have an eight o'clock curfew? But that's the stuff I dealt with, so if I wanted to go to a football game or something, I got questioned nine times about who was going to be there, what I was going to do, and who I was going to be with. So I avoided doing anything. I had an outgoing personality, so that wouldn't lead me into trouble as far as friends, but I was still one of The Princes.

Aunt Phyllis' quid pro quo was the Ten Commandments. Her modus operandi, her written law, was based on those edicts. "The Ten Commandments say, do not steal," she'd say. "The Ten Commandments say, honor your mother and your father." That was her big one: "Honor your mother, Chris."

Aunt Phyllis wasn't abusive, and I don't think that her punishments and things were done to scar me intentionally; she was what you might call a melodramatic diva. If someone does something very nice for me, but then say something hurtful about me, to me that is seriously conflicting. I think that if you love someone, you should never tear them down. But that behavior in Aunt Phyllis made a lot of people afraid of her.

Aunt Phyllis was something of a local power broker. She knew many high-profile people in the Democratic Party, including Jesse Jackson, all of the governors of North Carolina, and former President Bill Clinton. She was the kind of person, if you wanted to get anything done politically in Charlotte, you went to her for permission, especially if you were a minority, and double-especially if you were black. I witnessed a lot of those encounters with people who wanted Aunt Phyllis to do them a favor, and rather than rocking the boat, I just kind of went numb and did what I was told.

Aunt Phyllis would make fun of my smile. She would make fun of my personality, and that hit me to the core, because that's who I am—I'm happy, smiley, Chris. That's just me! I remember one time when she made this mocking smile to make fun of me, as if to say, "Oh Chris, stop doing that, you don't look real." She used to say that I was living a lie, but I was just a kid, you know? I got all this deep, deep shit thrown at me when I should have been crushing on girls and playing sports. So that's why church, youth group, and music were such oxygen to me. I would always escape into my headphones, because once I put the headphones on, all of that went away.

Now that I look back, I think part of my aunt's anger and frustration came from her diabetes. Momma Cille never had diabetes, but my grandfather Arthur did and Aunt Phyllis lost one of her legs. Momma Cille's Uncle Roscoe and my Aunt Thelma, Ma's sister, both lost a leg as well. When Aunt Thelma took us to mass, she'd have sugar packets in her purse for emergencies. One time Aunt Thelma had a sugar episode, and I saw her swallow four or five sugar packets during mass. I thought, "What the hell is going on?" Here I am, maybe nine or ten, seeing a person that I loved in a situation where I didn't even have a driver's license to take her somewhere if she got really sick. The last person that got diabetes in the family before I did was my Uncle Art.

I never saw my grandfather, or Aunt Thelma, or anyone, get upset because they had to deal with diabetes. They were always the kind of people who led a cause, who went from A to B for some kind of champion; who achieved victory for a cause, or for helping someone else. Diabetes was just part of the mix. Diabetes becoming a situation in people's lives was just, "Oh well, this is part of it. This is part of life."

I never heard them complain, and I always found that to be kind of noble, especially my grandfather. I never heard him talk about being tired. Now he would, you know, show it in his actions sometimes. He'd be snippy, or irritable, that kind of thing, but I never heard him complain. I never saw, or heard him even mention, fear and he never really stopped his habits, which were smoking cigarettes and cooking food with loads of fat and salt.

My grandfather, Arthur Patrick Lynch, Sr., was the rock of our family. He was the one who converted my grandmother and all her sisters to Catholicism. He was the quiet rock, in a good way, and he was the king of hospitality. What that meant was, if he met you for the first time, a meal was there and it would be a feast, almost in your honor. Usually, if he had enough time to prepare it, it would be exactly what you loved to eat. He would have found out your favorite foods, and tried to make them. Or, he would make a favorite dish of his to share with you. He would make red beans and rice, and what he called vermicelli—to this day I don't know exactly what it really was, but typically clams and spaghetti sauce were involved. I didn't like it, but it was something that everybody else would say, "Oh, that was great!" Because he was from Chicago, my grandfather was strictly a meat and potatoes guy, so it was always roast beef, steak and pork, including what Damion and I used to call "pig parts." Whenever we went to visit relatives up there, he would always make a stop up by Maxwell Street. They always had incredible food there, so he would be sure to go by and get the Polish sausages. My grandfather lived his life to the fullest. He was the king of smoking, the king of food; he loved his butter, and all the bad stuff, what makes your food taste good, he would use. But he was also the one who had coronary and diabetes issues.

To put it bluntly, we were the carb family. Carbs, carbs, and more carbs, before carbs were even talked about. Pastas, and the breads, and potatoes; all of that and more. Sweet tea was a staple in our house. Vegetables were really big in our family, too; you had to eat vegetables, but what offset the vegetables were carbohydrates. We had this tradition that we'd go out to dinner every Saturday after 5:30 mass. We'd either go to a place like Red Lobster, or the Hungry Fisherman, or this place that I still love in Charlotte called South 21. Everybody in our family was an incredible cook. So our meals were very rich and flavorful, and very southern, which meant that *everything* was fried. My grandfather loved to eat neck bones and rice, bacon, ham, and other fatty meats.

As we were growing up in elementary school he became diabetic, but this was back when diabetes treatment was not as advanced as it is today. Watching him test his urine at bath time made me afraid, and I would think, "I don't want to know what my sugar is in my blood and my urine." He was always drained and tired.

My grandfather never seemed to get control of his diabetes. In fact, he almost lost a limb. He didn't lose it in the end, but having that happen when both Aunt Phyllis and Aunt Thelma had lost limbs made me promise myself, "No. That will not be me." I knew in the back of my mind, though, that the abundance of this kind of food was not good. Plus, we'd eat a lot of fast food. There was a Hardee's restaurant near us, a Burger King, a McDonald's, and a Kentucky Fried Chicken—all within a few blocks. In fact, when I took my grandfather to get his last meal before he passed away after his heart attack, it was for fast food. I took him to get a combo meal at Kentucky Fried Chicken! It was weird, but he lived a good life; he lived a rich, life, full of friends and company, but he always suffered due to diabetes.

All along, on the inside, I had huge health fears. But another one of Momma Cille's mantras was, "I'm a warrior, not a worrier." So, if there were discussions about their struggles with diabetes, I was never privy to them. The logical side of me was saying, "I really want to know more about this struggle." But then I'd go back into fear. Fear has this way of giving you life; it was an unhealthy fuel, for my life, anyway.

One of the things that always made me very afraid was seeing a mother and a child hold each other. It bothered me at my core, and I know it was because I never would or never could do that with my own mother. The other thing that made me feel fear was receiving loving feedback from others, like my friends. We always hugged a lot at youth ministry events, but I never felt comfortable doing that, or knew what to do when someone told me they liked me, or that I was fun to be around. What could I say to that? I would just run away from it awkwardly. When I got older, I would mainly eat fast food. I didn't realize that eating a combo number two from Burger King was worse that smoking two packs of cigarettes a day, if you ate that two or three times a day. Yet, in the back of my mind, I sensed that at some point in time, diabetes was going to catch up to me. I never said the words, "I'm afraid I'll get diabetes" aloud to anyone. I saw my family members deal with their discomforts resulting from diabetes without changing their lives much. But that was unhealthy.

Dr. Jesse Craven was our family physician. He used to joke that out of all the Lynches, Momma Cille and I were the healthiest, because we never got the flu and rarely got sick. He said that we were destined to have the Big Ones. In our family, the Big Ones were high blood pressure, which I have; high cholesterol, which I have; and diabetes. While everybody else went through their diabetes control ups and downs, Dr. Craven said, "Chris, either you or Damion or both will get diabetes. It's just a matter of time." When he said that, I was like, "Oh, no!" All those fears in the back of my mind were just magnified, as if I were doomed.

The depression I often experienced in life, based on feelings of loss about my Mom, and other things, drove my reckless decisions about eating. I didn't do drugs; I didn't do alcohol. My vice was food.

3

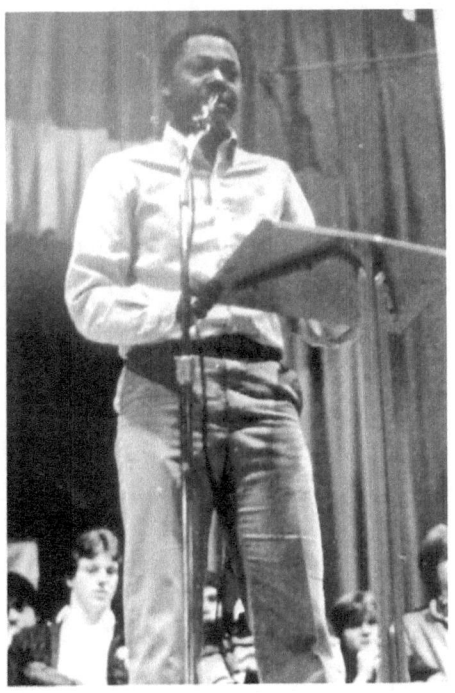

Catholic School

I learned about girls from Catholic School.

Once I became a teenager, I realized that I found Catholic women *hot*. St. Patrick Catholic School and Charlotte Catholic High School were where I learned about them—school uniforms, the whole fantasy. Growing up, it seemed the dudes I met always seemed to know so much more about girls then me. My romantic life for a long time was just that—fantasy. I remember dudes would say things like, "Yeah man, he's over there jacking off," and I would laugh with them, but I was too afraid to ask what they meant.

I was a big fan of Steve Martin in elementary and high school, and Aunt Phyllis got me an album of his for a present. He wrote a song about lesbians. When I listened to it and asked, "Hey, what's a lesbian?" Aunt Phyllis took the album away from me. I didn't find out what a lesbian was until much later!

Now I know, of course. Despite my lack of education in the sex department, though, my ratio of female-to-male friends was about 90:10. I had friends that were dudes, but I related better to women. That said, I was so afraid of the consequences of sex that I didn't even masturbate. I *wanted* to date, I wanted to French kiss, I wanted to do all of those things, and I had opportunities, but I chose not to capitalize on them because of my fear. Over the past several years I've reconnected with many of my friends from those schools, and some of the women have said that they had crushes on me in high school. But I was completely oblivious about their feelings at the time.

Back in the day we had all this crazy-colored clothing—fuchsia, chartreuse, you know, that Flashdance look?—and it was just a happy time. Sixth through eighth grade at St. Pat's, and my years at Charlotte Catholic High School were ecstasy. I love those times and I still vibe on them today.

The girls were preppy, wearing little short skirts and little heels, and oh, that was so hot. The movies I watch to bring back my memories of those times are ones like *Valley Girl* and *Fast Times at Ridgemont High*. Those days were, and are still, sacred days. I joke with my Charlotte Catholic friends that our school days were like Fast Times at Charlotte Catholic High, but without the surfers.

One good friend, who I'll call Darlene, was one of the high school girls that I remember walking to class and kissing. Our tongues touched, and I had wood the entire time! But looking back, I can see that fear was crippling me. I could have hung out, dated and even gotten laid, and I think I would have calmed down way earlier in life. The turbulent hurdles I faced, trying to get up to 40,000 feet of happiness, would not have been as bumpy. I wouldn't have spilled soda and water and everything all over; I would have been flying first class, probably a lot of it in the mile-high club!

It's funny when I look back on it now, but you know, I was never a pig. When girls would break up with their boyfriends, they'd come to me for solace. These women would tell me everything, because I wasn't trying to sleep with them or otherwise take advantage. I have to tell you, though, sometimes I would want to, and be totally bummed because I fell into the friend zone when I wanted to be in the freak zone!

I always had what the dudes called groupies, and there's some juicy stuff in my yearbooks. Girls would write messages like, "Oh Chris, you're so hot," "You're sexy," and "I just love you." But I never equated that with an opportunity for getting laid. I remember one girl who wrote to me, "I love it when you hold me and touch me." Momma Cille read that and said, "Oh my, Chris, this one called you sexy!" I just said something like, "Alright, that's cool." But I would never have done anything about those hints.

I didn't realize I had a nuclear bomb that I could have ignited with many, many women. I remember when I left as a senior at Charlotte Catholic, women *cried*. "Chris is leaving, oh My God!" I'm sitting there thinking, "Why are they crying? What in the world are they so upset about?" Instead of thinking that, though, I should have been saying, "That's okay, dear. Come over here and let me say goodbye to you properly."

Today, even though my Kryptonite is controlling women, I trust women more than men. If you look at scripture, the men always screwed Jesus over, but the women were the faithful ones. Yet, in high school and the first years of college, whenever I was aware of a kinetic energy happening between me and a woman, I never thought I was good enough to take it to the next level.

Being at a Catholic high school, the church was integrated into my life, but not in an over-bearing or repressive way. Diocesan high schools naturally took part in pretty much every program that the Office of Youth Ministry put together. Besides all the time I spent at school and playing in church, some of my nights and weekends involved Catholic youth activities. The Diocese of Charlotte had a vibrant, active ministry for its youth, and the get-togethers often brought me into close contact with people from all over the western half of North Carolina. They also brought me closer to my Charlotte Catholic friends.

There were retreats held at parishes and at the Diocesan Youth Center in Flat Rock, which maintained a house on the grounds of Our Lady of the Hills campground. During the summer, Our Lady of the Hills was a Catholic summer camp for younger kids, but for the other nine months, it was usually ours when there weren't boy scout outings there.

The youth ministry office held weekend retreats for small groups of kids, and parish youth groups could also hold retreats there. All the Catholic schools held retreats there as well. There were fall and winter retreats where you could learn to climb and participate in trust activities, freeze your tail off while you were singing the "Glory and Praise" songs, and pray huddled together in huge blankets for body warmth. The crowning jewel of youth ministry activities was the yearly spring Diocesan Youth Conference, where kids from all over the diocese camped out in tents, held workshops, and gave talks. We had huge masses that would take hours because giving the peace sign to one another took forever. At most Roman Catholic services, giving one another a sign of Christ's peace involves a handshake and a kind word, but at youth ministry masses, you received full-body hugs from everyone. I remember attending several retreats where the sign of peace was postponed until the end of the mass, so the attending priest could take a break and not have to stand waiting at the altar while we all hugged everybody else there for 20 or 30 minutes.

At the youth conferences, I hung out with my friends from St. Pat's and Charlotte Catholic, and whomever else I knew from other churches. I always brought my guitar, and we'd have informal sing-alongs and jam sessions all the time. Some of my happiest memories are being together with those friends—singing, laughing, telling outrageous stories, and talking about God and prayer in a real, meaningful way.

In Flat Rock, nobody wore uniforms — it was jeans and shirts, buttons, face paint, rainbow trousers and crazy hats. I became known for wearing this one blue ball cap, and people said they could tell it was me from even far away if they heard a guitar, saw the cap, and saw a huge group of girls. Back then, my smiles were real, and I was at peace.

Momma Cille was the Matriarch. She was the Teacher, the Mother, the Grandmother. Ma controlled what I did and how I did it. I know now that she did it out of love for me, but when I was growing up I didn't separate her love from her control. There was a high expectation level that I put on myself to be the person she wanted me to be, and in fact, I lived most of my life with very strong, dominant, controlling women telling me what to do. The pressure that I put on myself was probably my interpretation of her reaction to life.

"No cross, no crown," was the way that she operated. It's like she had that old school Southern grandmother role down pat. She had enough love to give to everybody, but some people were on her "list." God help you if you were on it.

I was a B minus, C student. I could have been a 4.0 student, but I didn't challenge myself to be. I really sucked at math and science, but was good at history, English and religion, which intrigued me enough to become a theology major in college. I had my challenges academically, but I think most of them stemmed from low self-esteem. Momma Cille would put scathing messages on my report cards, as if she was blaming my teachers for my poor performance. Once in seventh or eighth grade I had a D in a class, and Ma wrote back to the teacher, "If we don't get this fixed, I'll take him out of school." To her, that was a serious threat, and it scared me, too, because I loved being at Catholic school.

I wish now that I had cut loose of my fear of failure while in high school. If I had, I think I would have been more academically disciplined when I enrolled at Belmont Abbey College in 1984.

Did I mention that Ma's prejudice, if she had any, was that if you were Catholic, you were practically sinless? She was relieved and proud when both Damion and I chose to go to Belmont Abbey. The Abbey was not my first choice, however. I actually had my heart set on going to a larger school, like the University of Notre Dame, or Penn State. Belmont Abbey is a small Catholic liberal arts college north of Charlotte, maintained by the Benedictine monks of Mary Help of Christians Abbey.

We were very familiar with the Abbey. In 1972, the Abbey went co-ed, and when Damion arrived there eleven years later, one dorm was actually co-ed, too, although of course men and women did not share rooms. The Abbey was small enough that pretty much everyone knew what you were up to, literally; if you really kicked up your heels, you were likely to be the named subject of the sermon at the student's mass on Sunday night.

Momma Cille dropped me off at the Abbey, and before she left she said, "Chris, I am so proud of you." I could see her relief that I was at another Catholic school, because to her that was the safest place for me. I needed that moment, and it meant a lot that she gave it to me. Being at college was a bit scary at first, but not as frightening as I imagined it would have been at one of the bigger schools. If I had gone to one of those, I would have been completely alone, and I was in far too much fear to do something like that.

I had been visiting Damion all throughout his freshman year, and had gotten to know the guys he hung out with, so I had a built-in group of friends at the Abbey. Once again, most of my activities were built around church, in that our core group of friends went to five o'clock mass almost every weekday, and sometimes went to sing Vespers at seven p.m. It was us and the monks jamming out!

At the Abbey, I continued my explorations into sound and music. My room was full of rock posters, with several of my main man, Eddie Van Halen, and I had a kick-ass stereo setup. My friends would ask for my help with their stereo systems after they heard mine. Of course, I would always modify the equipment in some way with my electronic gadgets.

Each dorm room at the Abbey was equipped with wooden desks and shelves that were attached to the wall. This was before subwoofers, so to get great bass response, I turned my speakers on their sides, because wood amplifies sound greatly. I often make a joke that you know you've hooked up your stereo rig correctly when somebody yells at you, "Hey, turn that damned thing down!" I turned my desk area into the stereo cabinet, so I heard that a lot.

At the Abbey, I saw how my friends were doing well on their own, making grades, and some of my friends were working at jobs at the same time to be able to afford spending time doing what they wanted to do, which I admired. When one of my friends left to go to work, I'd envy them. I wanted to do that, to make my own money, but if I said that to Ma, she'd have practically killed me. "You can't go to school and work at the same time," was what she would have said.

When most people were getting laid and going to parties on the weekends, Damion and I had to go home. I remember one weekend I did stay on campus, and I had a blast. It was so fun to be away from home, but doing that weekly would have been taboo. Ma said, "Now don't do that every weekend!" And the guilt would come in. I never had a girlfriend who lived at the Abbey, either. I wanted to, so badly, but I didn't allow myself to form those kinds of relationships, to be together with just one person.

The one that I was the closest to at the Abbey was Mike. I met him before I got there one Friday afternoon when I came up to visit Damion. Mike came in to his room—they were living in the same suite of rooms together—and he was wearing this ugly-ass Japanese-looking robe. He had the old Neil Peart look, too—long hair and a mustache. He just sat down and said "Hi, I'm Mike," and we bonded fast. We immediately started talking about music, and he got me listening to all the Canadian bands like Rush and Triumph. He was from Minnesota, and being closer to Canada, he first caught that stuff from the radio.

Mike played drums, and he idolized Peart. We would hang out in his room listening to music, and I would play air guitar with a pick while he'd play air drums with sticks. That's how we learned our chops so when we got into a band situation we knew each other's signals. Mike came over to St. Patrick's for Saturday night mass, and eventually he started playing with the folk group. To this day, Damion, Mike and I always have this constant running laugh track together, no matter what we're doing or where we are, and after being apart for a bit, we pick up right where we left off. That is our chemistry.

Mike is my band mate for life, and I have some of the most electrical memories of music connection with him, Damion and my friend Don. Mike and I could get together with Damion tomorrow and play a set, and we'd probably play something from the Who or Boston. Mike and I have talked about girls, rock and roll, life, ups, downs—we cried together, even. He and I are just blood. We still catch shows together whenever we can.

We'd talk about women and what we wanted. I could get explicit with him, and he'd reciprocate and give me ideas on how to handle sexual situations and girls. I'd get frustrated though, because I wanted to do all these things but was inhibited, whereas he would go do them. He was hanging from the chandeliers, and I was watching him realizing, "Hey, you can hang on chandeliers—awesome!" But he executed. I'll just leave it at that.

Near the end of my sophomore year, a woman I'm going to call Mary joined the folk group. She was a very natural acoustic guitar player. James Taylor was her big influence of hers, and I loved how she played her D chords the way he did. I always respected the acoustic players that could get a unique sound, because I'm power, and metal, and to get rock effects like that you have to add electronics. Acoustic players get their sound just from the way they pick and strum.

As I entered my junior year, I could feel my life changing. It was as if my cocoon started cracking open. Mary was going through her own transformation, where she was separated from her husband then divorced, and then going through an annulment process. Emotionally, I was becoming a wreck. I began to struggle in my classes, and my prayer life was becoming combative. I would sit in the silence and just agonize with God about what to do with myself, because I was not happy at school or with anything I was learning in the theology department. I was growing up and realizing I wanted something different from my life. My classes were actually boring, because I had heard so much of what was being taught at Charlotte Catholic. I wasn't excited by theological discussions like my other friends in the program were. I felt like the odd man out all the time.

Mary would come over to the Abbey to visit after work and hang out, and we'd have many conversations before she left in the parking lot. She was lonely, and I was lonely and feeling pulled away from the Abbey. I felt I needed to jump into life, not stay in school, and school was not working out. As the spring semester of 1987 approached, I was feeling as if an event as big as my confirmation, or going to that Van Halen concert, was about to happen. Mary was seven years older than me and a professional woman who was dressed up all the time and seemed to be free of the obligations I had. With her being Catholic and playing in the folk group with us, I felt nudged towards her, a nudge that I'm going to call a divine nudge, something that said, "Chris, this is your time." God was giving me my 40 days in the desert. Everything that I had relied on so much before now was just not helping.

My grades were plummeting. I was going through many internal conflicts, like struggling with self-esteem, and man stuff, and I didn't have a father figure to talk to about the way I was feeling. Fears and questions were colliding inside me. I couldn't concentrate on anything but the pain and angst I felt, and everything I tried to do academically fell apart. I wasn't learning and growing, I was just floundering. I felt like I was imploding while everything around me was exploding, and I couldn't figure out how to stop it.

I felt like I had become "Chris, blank." I felt like I had interchangeable nouns after my name: Damion's brother, Lucille's grandson, or Phyllis' nephew. The worst was being Damion's brother, because I didn't make friends of my own; all my Abbey friends knew Damion before me. I started to despise being called that. Damion and I talked about it many years later, and he apologized for it, but that feeling wasn't his fault. I was just tired of being his shadow on campus. I wanted freedom, and self-worth; I wanted to have my own identity independent from my family.

Eventually I was called in for a conversation with the head of the theology department, and he told me I simply had to get my academics up or I wasn't going to make it to my senior year. But the Abbey was beginning to have less and less importance in my life. Besides the bad grades I was getting, my grandfather's death the previous year had hit me harder than I realized. I didn't remember my Mother dying, so my grandfather's death was my first crushing loss. Suddenly getting a college degree didn't matter anymore. I wanted to get a life degree.

At the same time, Momma Cille's over-protective love was weighing me down. She would always say things in a fearful way—you know, don't do this thing because other bad things will happen— not to humiliate me or make me feel bad, but because that was her way of showing love. I really wanted to fall and scrape my knees like my friends were doing, with self-reliance. I wanted to feel normal, but I felt like I was drowning under her.

Ma saw my grades and she must have noticed how I was detaching. Whenever any of her children did anything that she didn't see as in their best interest, she would jump in and assume the position of control. Instead of Ma sitting me down and saying, "Chris, I know you've got a lot going on right now. Why don't we talk about it?" she got mad at me. I wonder now if she didn't know how to deal with that kind of thing, because Aunt Phyllis and I had a similar situation when I was a little kid.

Aunt Phyllis was taking me to school, and I was having a bad, emotional day. Rain was falling as hard as my tears. I don't know why I was crying, but I know I could not articulate it and say, "I'm miserable, I'm unhappy, I miss my Mom." Aunt Phyllis had a jar of change in her car, and she rummaged in there and handed me a quarter, as if to say, "Here's something. I don't know how to fix you, or help you." I'm sure she left frustrated that day. When I walked into St. Pat's, I felt completely alone. Her and Momma Cille's thing was to confront you sideways by going above your head and having some other authority bring you to face it. That's how they dealt with difficult things.

So I found out that Momma Cille wanted to set me straight when the President of the Abbey called me into his office. Now, this wasn't as big of a deal as you might think. The Abbey was a small place, and you could talk to any faculty or staff member easily. All of the classrooms and offices were in two buildings barely twenty steps apart, so we were all familiar with everyone we encountered. Even the front desk secretary knew every student's name. The monastery was connected to those buildings as well, and though you couldn't go through the doors that led to the monk's rooms, there was really no separation between life and work for them, or us. Their life was educating and ministering to students, and they did it where they lived. We saw them night and day, and the doors were usually open. The other faculty and staff members' doors were as well.

I knew, of course, that the President wanted to talk about my academic performance, because my G.P.A. was so low the college was going to have to take action, and probably suspend me. But I didn't realize that he was going to affirm everything I felt. He told me that my grandmother had asked him to talk to me about my academic performance, but he didn't feel comfortable scolding me like a child. This was one of his students sitting in front of him, and he wanted to find out what was going on inside.

He said to me, "It probably bugs the hell out of you that you're always referred to as Damion's brother." I lied to him and told him it didn't, but I wanted to cry, because he hit the nail right on the head. As we talked, I knew he really understood how I felt. Even though I walked out of there knowing that if I didn't step up, I was going to be out of college, I felt that I had a chance to do something else worthwhile. Here was someone that saw something in me.

As he was talking to me, I realized how numb I had become to my pain. In therapy, years later, I used an analogy to describe how I felt that last semester at the Abbey. Imagine taking your hand and putting it into a vise grip, then cranking down on it so hard that you reach a point where there is no pain. If somebody then released that vise grip off, your hand would still feel numb even though it was broken. That's what I felt like.

As I walked from his office back to my dorm room, I saw Mike. He was sitting on the ledge outside of my door with this look of peace and inclusion. He belonged there, but I was coming apart inside. I realized that I didn't want to stay there anymore. It wasn't that I didn't love all of my friends and enjoy hanging out with them, but I was being pulled away. I knew that the road was going to be long, and I didn't even know if I even had the right tires on the car to drive down it. I was deep in the woods.

I went to St. Patrick's, which had always been a happy place for me. I knelt in one of the front pews and I prayed for God to give me the courage to leave. One of the sisters in the school passed through who I knew well, but she knew me as the person I had been, and I couldn't be that anymore. I told myself, "When I leave here, I will not be the same." God seemed to be saying something to me that sounded like, "Chris, it's time to go. Leave the Abbey." So I dropped out of school.

I didn't lose Mike. He graduated that year, and decided to stay in Charlotte to start a career. He joined the folk group and played drums with Damion and me, and we got tighter. The bad part was that I had to make my new life without the resources I had previously. For example, there was some money that was left over in my account at the Abbey that should have come back to me, but Momma Cille had my access to it revoked. It seemed as if she wanted me to suffer. I understand now that she wanted me to feel the full brunt of my decision. Luckily I had spent so much time at Reliable Music, buying stuff for my rig and playing guitar, that I knew all the sales people well. So when I wanted to get a job, it was easy to get one there. Of course Momma Cille didn't like it; she was not impressed. My first job, and earning my first minimum wage paycheck, happened without her and Aunt Phyllis having anything to do with it.

Not only had I left the Abbey, but soon thereafter Mary and I got hot and heavy, and I moved in with her. To Aunt Phyllis and Ma, doing those things was simply irresponsibility bordering on immorality. They considered my life to be opposite from the way that they had raised me. Damion never changed his opinion of me though; never. He always respected my choices. Aunt Phyllis wouldn't even talk to me, and Ma and I were not in the best relationship. Ma did not approve of my choices, and some of the nastiest, hurtful moments she and I ever had together happened during this time.

For my part, I jumped into this new life—sex, work, bills and everything that went with independence. Mike and I became like brothers, and he and Damion became really close, too. Mary gave me permission to be the sexual Chris, and there was definitely a maturation process that came as a result. I was a late bloomer and had some catching up to do. I was drawn to her because she was already out in the world, making money and living her life. Whenever I was around her I would feel exhilarated.

Ma let me know that I was living in sin every opportunity she had. She would call down to the music store and kind of harass me. There was a joke Damion and I would make about her when she got into that mode. We called it the Wrath. For example, we'd never be late even two minutes for anything, because the Wrath was not worth it. Mary and I had turmoil because of our age difference, and we didn't have the same goals, and eventually it ended. When Mary's marriage was finally annulled, I didn't want to marry her. The day that I broke up with Mary, Ma was relieved. Happily relieved.

Eventually working at Reliable Music ran its course, and I took the opportunity to go work at GE Capital. GE only lasted about a year, but that was okay, because I really wanted to be in sales. A medical salesman I met through Mary became one of my mentors at that time, and I looked up to him a lot.

Besides being independent, my secondary goal was to live in ZIP code 28226, which was South Charlotte where all my friends in high school had lived. My sales mentor was a guy who had it all—cash, cars and a hot wife. He was my Gordon Gekko, and he taught me everything I know about sales. He would cut through the training seminar lines and say very basic, very real things that helped me understand what sales is really about. He'd say there's a way to get through to people, but you can't get there by being a bullshitter. Or, in his words, "Nobody gives a fuck about you, so you have to give them a reason to."

I got work as a hospital buyer, which was my initial workplace training to be a sales representative, since I worked with salespeople all day. To get the buyer job, I should have had a college degree, so I started what I call now my uphill climb, a period in my life that lasted more than ten years where I felt I was raking water uphill. To get the life I thought I wanted, I had to sell myself before I could sell anything else. Today people I work with say I'm a guy that knows how to close, but it took a good while to get here.

I had to meet with the guy who would be my boss three times before he agreed to hire me. The third time he said I was too good to be true, so he had needed to double check me before he made a mistake. He said, "You've got everything you need except a college degree." But once I got in I did a great job, and was able to move into medical sales, which I did for about four years. During this time frame, I went through a layoff and I met my wife.

4

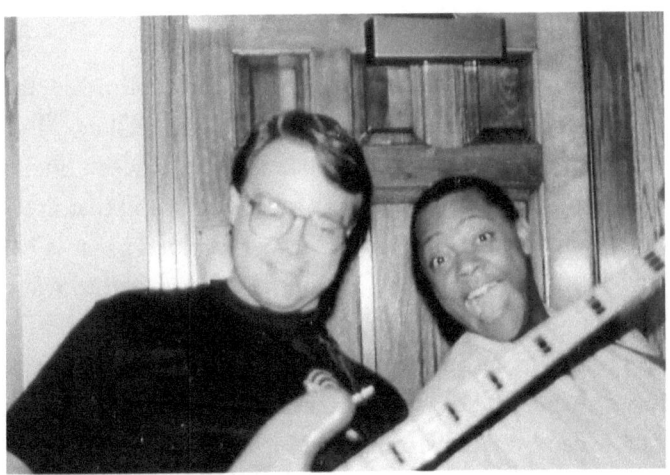

Intensive Care

"You're black, you're over 40, you have
high blood pressure and high cholesterol,
and now you have severe diabetes.

The next thing for you is a stroke."

Dr. Kamath, my night doctor, was explaining to me exactly what my body was dealing with and the realities of my situation. I had come in to the hospital thinking I was just dehydrated, and I wanted to believe that was all that was wrong with me. But Dr. Kamath had nipped that line of thinking in the bud by telling me that death was still not out of the question.

"Chris," he said to me plainly, "Here's your situation. We're trying several things, and by process of elimination we'll figure out how to treat you."

When I heard "try," I had to stop him from going further. "Wait a minute," I said, "you don't know how to treat this?"

"No. Your blood sugar is all over the place, and we don't know how to treat it. There is no known way to do it."

Earlier that day when I heard Dr. Kishan, the daytime doctor, tell me that I was moving in the right direction, I thought, "Okay, I'll just go to sleep now." I was going in and out—passing out, I guess. She said what they were mostly concerned about were my kidneys, and that my heart was "very irritable and erratic." I heard her say, "His blood sugar is 1400," and later, "Now 1100." So whatever they did initially started to work. Then I remember being whisked away to intensive care.

When I heard "intensive care," I got a pit in my stomach. They took me to the intensive care unit (ICU) on my gurney. One of my favorite shows used to be "Emergency" when I was growing up, and I felt like I was at Rampart Hospital being whisked around, with all the tubes and the electrodes being placed on me for the EKG, and oxygen. I had intravenous bags hanging on me, several of them. One bag was to hydrate me and one bag was insulin. I had an IV in my right arm for so long when I was there that I can still bend it to this day and feel where the needle was. I had an IV in my left hand on the other side.

I remember all of those things being placed on me, feeling the nastiness and smell of medical chemicals. The kits and the adhesives and my personal favorite, isopropyl alcohol—not! I hate that. Oh, and I had the oxygen tube blowing in my nose. Then I started feeling someone poking around Mr. Happy, and realized they were putting a catheter in me.

I felt that sharp pain, and I'm like, "Un-huh! No way, dude!" The male nurse said, "Mr. Lynch, you'll pee on yourself." I said, "I'll take that risk, no problem. I don't want that damned catheter in me."

So he yanked it out! The pain of that coming out of my penis, that sensation, was *so* nasty. But even with all the poking and prodding and stuff that they did to me in the ICU at Carolinas Medical Center-Pineville, I was treated with the utmost of beautiful care and excellence, which I needed desperately. You know what they say on "ER" all the time when someone is critical? "He's coding?" All my alarms were going off; I was coding.

There was fluid in my chest cavity, leaking from my swelling heart. I was put on a Cardizem drip to prevent me from going into arrest so I would not have a heart attack. Besides the swelling in my chest, my EKG had come back looking as if a little kid had drawn in the lines upside down.

When you see one of those EKG readings on TV demonstrating a heart rate, you see a pattern I'm sure everyone is familiar with: there's a real sharp, tall line going up and a very short line going down. When I received my medical records later and took a look at the reading, it was like my EKG line was backwards. I had a very tiny short line going up and a really long one going down. So the chemical and electrical feedback that goes on in your heart that basically keeps your blood moving—while your heart is pumping, there's also electrical reaction going on in your blood from your brain that's telling it to move the heart, telling the blood to move—was not happening. My battery was drained, and I was extremely close to brain death. I could have had a stroke.

The trauma that my body was going through was catastrophic, but I was not the only one suffering. After I arrived in my ICU room, Momma Cille and Blanche came in, and when Momma Cille saw me lying up in there, I think she had another motherly moment. She was always a fighter, and she got through some terrible things, but this shocked her. This was one of those moments when I really felt her love for me, because Ma was scared, but all she could think of was what to do for me next. I was in and out of sleep because basically there was a war going on inside of my body. With all these fluids coming in, my kidneys were shutting on, off, off, on; my pancreas was sputtering—it just was a mess.

I remember saying, "Blanche, please call Don. Here's his number."

When I left Reliable Music in 1988, which was a music store I had practically lived in for most of my life, I went to work for GE Capital, and that's where I met Donald Russell.

I was what was called a re-marketing specialist. That basically meant I was repossessing homes. Oh God, talk about tragedy in the real estate world! I was "repo"-ing mobile homes and refurbishing them for resale at lots in the southeast. Which meant the company would go get a repo'd mobile home, put money in it to fix it up, and then resell it.

That was my first example of working in big corporate America. I had to wear a suit every day and was around all these hot women who were all dressed up, and it was just—I was in heaven. I was standing at the copy machine one day and Don came up to use it, and we started talking about music, and he said, "Oh, I'm a bass player." And I'm like, "Well I'm a guitar player." Then I asked him *the question*, which is seriously important for any musician. You can always tell a real musician from their influences. So I asked Don, "Who's your influence on bass guitar?"

He answered, "Well, who's yours on guitar?"

"Mine's Eddie Van Halen, and Jimi Hendrix," I said, "You know, Johnny Cash, B.B. King, and those guys."

Don said, "Mine's Jaco Pastorius."

My mouth dropped, cause Jaco is a—I mean, he's dead now, but he is a *beyond* bass player. That's when I knew Don was serious about playing, and from that moment it was like a light hit the copy machine and the angels started singing "Alleluia!" I knew we'd bond, and 20 or more years later, he and I are still tight. He was in the legal department, so whenever the repo thing didn't work out to where we could refurbish them for re-sale, Don was working to get stuff in line so GE could get covered in their losses. About a year or so later, both of us got laid off and moved on, but we have remained best friends.

Don does not take no for an answer. He will tell you to fuck off if necessary, but it will be in the chivalrous way of a Southern gentleman—a very genteel gentleman.

The staff at the hospital gave him some problems in the beginning, and Don said to them in his very old-school, Southern manner, "I'm Donald, son of David, and I'm here to see Christopher Lynch."

They asked, "Are you related to him?"

He said, "I am Don, his best friend. I am going to see my best friend. Where is he?" He got very insistent. As he would recount to me later, "That is not a question, that is not an option; I am going to see him. So thank you. You're *recused*."

They let him in.

I had asked Blanche to call Don, and then went back to sleep. The next thing I remember is Don bursting into the ICU, and I go, "Hey man!"

There are a few people in life that refer to me as Christopher: Don, and my friends Lauren, Kelly, and Valerie. Aunt Phyllis and Ma called me Christopher because my Mom wanted me to be called Christopher, not Chris, which is kind of funny because I like Chris way better. Later on in life, Momma Cille started calling me Chris. Don calls me "Christopher, yo!"

I think he wasn't expecting to see what he saw in the ICU, because after he said yo, he said, "Wow!"

And I said, "Yeah, Don, I'm pretty fucked up." I was saying bad words in front of Momma Cille! But I thought, "You know what, I'm butt-ass vulnerable naked now, so I'm just going to be the authentic me. I'm not going to mince words; I'm just putting it out there." I wasn't grumpy—I was always pleasant to everyone—but I was scared.

Don recognized that, and he basically took over for me. He said, "Chris, I got it." Kind of like in the Gospels, when Jesus told John to take care of Mary and he just went and did it without question? Don and I always have biblical reference jokes.

I said something to the effect of, "Don, please take care of Momma Cille. I feel like shit," and I fell asleep again.

Ma was very nervous. I knew that because she kept talking about the past, telling the same stories over and over. Don was the recipient of that. People normally see me happy and up and the life of the party, but I was laying there dying, or coming out of death, or whatever it was I was in the midst of, and everybody freaked out.

With all the people coming in the room, I told the nurses, "There's going to be a lot of people coming to see me that don't look like me, but if they say they're here to see me and they're family, it's OK."

They asked, "What do you mean?"

I told them, "They're all white, except Ma, Blanche and a few other people."

Don pretty much was on watch with Momma Cille and Blanche until they left to go over to Tony Roma's to get something to eat. Only Don was left in the hospital room with me, and although I was in and out of consciousness I remember Don told me, "Chris, just convalesce. Heal."

About an hour and a half later, Ma came back with takeout from Tony Roma's. All the meters attached to me started going off the charts because I could smell the acidity in those ribs. They smelled great, yet the smell was painful to me. When you're in the hospital and all that purity is flowing into you, that kind of food is toxic. So I said, "Ma! Get that shit out of here!"

Don said, "Come on Momma Cille; let me run this down to your car." I remember him taking the box out of there. The people that I remember visiting me were Paul and Tom, my neighbors, with Tom's wife Barb; Don; Seanta, my friend from elementary school; and Blanche, Momma Cille, Tony, and Tony's wife Yvonne.

Don called Damion and said, "Damion, your brother's dying." Don knew what was happening because he had spoken with my doctors, and he tried to explain to my brother what was going on. Nobody thought I was going to make it.

Some of the very first orders Dr. Kishan gave were for how much insulin to administer to me. In my medical charts there is a copy of the insulin regimen recommended to bring a person's blood level under control. It is in a section of my insulin orders entitled "Corrective / Supplemental Insulin Scales," and there are three separate tables listing insulin dose algorithms and how to calculate them. When I was admitted, Dr. Kishan and her staff could not determine if I had Type I or Type II diabetes, but that didn't matter as much as figuring out how to bring my blood glucose to a safe level. The tables looked like this:

Low Dose Algorithm		Moderate Dose Algorithm		High Dose Algorithm	
Thin, elderly, or renal patient, or total daily insulin requirement below 35 units		Average size ptient or total daily insulin requirement 35-60 units		Very insulin resistant, or septic patient, or total daily insulin requirement more than 60 units	
Scale for TIDAC*, Q4H**, and Q6H**		Scale for TIDAC, Q4H, and Q6H		Scale for TIDAC, Q4H, and Q6H	
Blood Glucose	Additional insulin	Blood Glucose	Additional insulin	Blood Glucose	Additional insulin
Below 70	Follow hypoglycemia orders	Below 70	Follow hypoglycemia orders	Below 70	Follow hypoglycemia orders
70-120	zero units	70-120	zero units	70-120	zero units
121-170	1 units	121-150	1 units	121-135	1 units
171-220	2 units	151-180	2 units	136-150	2 units
221-270	3 units	181-210	3 units	151-165	3 units
271-320	4 units	211-240	4 units	166-180	4 units
321-370	5 units	241-270	5 units	181-195	5 units
Over 370	6 units	271-300	6 units	196-210	6 units
		301-330	7 units	211-225	7 units
		331-160	8 units	226-240	8 units
		Over 360	10 units	241-255	9 units
				256-270	10 units
				271-285	11 units
				286-300	12 units
				301-315	13 units
				316-330	14 units
				Over 330	15 units
Scale for QHS**** and 2 AM		Scale for QHS and 2 AM		Scale for QHS and 2 AM	
Blood Glucose	Additional insulin	Blood Glucose	Additional insulin	Blood Glucose	Additional insulin
Below 70	Follow hypoglycemia orders	Below 70	Follow hypoglycemia orders	Below 70	Follow hypoglycemia orders
70-140	zero units	70-140	zero units	70-140	zero units
141-190	1 units	141-170	1 units	141-170	2 units
191-240	2 units	171-230	3 units	171-200	4 units
241-290	3 units	231-290	5 units	201-230	6 units
Over 290	4 units	Over 290	6 units	231-290	8 units
				Over 290	10 units

*TIDAC (t.i.d, a.c.)=Three times a day, before meals
**Q4H=Every four hours
***Q6H=Every six hours
****QHS=At bedtime

They selected a high dose algorithm, which was indicated for "insulin resistant or septic" patients. Sepsis is a condition in which all of your organs become so infected they begin to die one by one. I wasn't septic, but I was severely acidotic, and my body had to get enough insulin so that it would burn glucose (sugar) for energy instead of fat. This would allow my blood cells to become healthy again. The highest blood glucose level listed in the tables is "over 330," and my blood glucose was almost five times that. Dr. Kishan ordered that I be given ten units of insulin initially, 20 units when I arrived in ICU, and then eight more units each hour. That was the Chris Lynch insulin scale.

Besides diabetic ketoacidosis—the point at which one's blood becomes acidotic—I was hypothermic and suffering from some sort of infection. That was what had made me feel like I had the flu. I was also diagnosed with the following conditions when I entered the hospital:

- **Hyperkalemia**, or an extremely high potassium level that can be fatal as it causes arrhythmia, or irregular heartbeat.
- **Hyperlipidemia**, or abnormally high rates of fat in the blood.
- **Hypertension**, or high blood pressure.
- **Atrial fibrillation with rapid ventricular response** (RVR), or irregular electrical activity in the heart, which can cause rapid heartbeat.
- **Severe metabolic acidosis**, or an excessive amount of acid in bodily fluids, which causes rapid breathing, anxiety, mental confusion and fatigue.
- **Gastrointestinal/deep venous thrombosis prophylaxis**, which is the presence of a blood clot blocking the gastrointestinal tract.

I remember a heavy, warm blanket being put on me, and tubes and beeping, and people moving all around me. You know when people talk about "hitting rock bottom?" To me, what I went through is about as close as I think anyone could come to being on the cross, because I was totally dependent on other people, and every part of my person, down to my bodily fluids, was up for inspection. I was also as naked as a baby, because they had to get my clothes off me to dress me in the flattering hospital robes that everyone was wearing that season. When my clothes came off, I still had my socks on, and that's when I was introduced to my hospital robe. It was me, my athletic socks, and a white robe with huge armholes.

When I get scared, humor calms me. I think of funny things and I try to laugh. Even though this was the part where I was facing death, I was still me in the midst of it—making jokes. When they moved me to ICU, I realized I didn't have my underwear on. The first nurse I saw in ICU was really hot, and I knew I had to have underwear on. I was thinking, "These women are too fine! My wood will really stick up—I've got to have something on." So I found my underwear in a bag with my other clothes, and I put them on.

A nurse in the ICU asked me several questions to admit me as a patient into the hospital. They asked me about my vaccinations and such. I told them I had not had a flu shot, so she told me I could get one there. I don't know why, but I refused the shot. Given how many times I was poked, prodded and stuck in the next several days, this fact, listed in my medical records, never fails to make me crack up now.

Now you know I had to do everything first class; my first time to the hospital and I don't go to a regular room, I'm in the damned ICU! Since I had refused the catheter, I didn't get the luxury of not worrying about having to pee. But I had what felt like fifty bags of fluid going into me, so I had to go. Here comes my first comedy routine for the ICU audience.

You now that little container they give men to pee in that little jug thing? I'm sitting there thinking, "I don't need a nurse for this! I just need to piss in this jug thing." So I'm sitting there pissing, and all of a sudden I feel this flood. I pissed all over myself!

The nurse comes in and starts laughing at me. She goes, "Mr. Lynch, give me that thing."

. I'm going, "What the?" She patiently explained that I had used the jug upside-down. I looked at her and said, in a very small voice, "Help me."

I think my good relationship with my nurses began then, because they thought, "This guy is a funny guy. He's peeing in the jug upside down!" They all start laughing, and I'm laughing at myself for doing it, because I had taken the jug sitting on the nurses' cart, and was sitting there singing to myself, "Oh, doo-dah, doo-dah, it's me, Chris, just doing what comes naturally!" and suddenly I realized, "Oh shit, that feels warm! Oh no! I just peed all over myself!" Instantly we all bonded.

When you're in intensive care, with all that movement and buzzing, you can't forget that they monitor absolutely everything. They took so many fluids from me, at one point the joke that I made was, "You're taking everything, do you want sperm with that? Do you want spit? You're stealing every fluid of mine, are you sure you don't want anything else?

The night nurse told me she had gone to school at the University of North Carolina in Chapel Hill, which was great because I'm a Tarheel fan. I think she was Russian, and she was really, really cool. She was serious, but had a great sense of humor, too. She said to me, "Chris, you need a wife."

I said, "Exactly! You got any friends? Hook me up! Let's talk about girls; that will get my mind off the IV." She loved that.

As I gradually became more aware of what was going on, basically my blood was waking up again and I started feeling a very little bit better. Being stuck in the bed was driving me nuts. Still, I was a very sick Chris. I could walk and I could stand, but they didn't want me to urinate in the toilet. They wanted me to pee in the jug so they could check the level of ketones in my urine.

I got very fidgety; I think I was trying to pretend I wasn't terrified. As I remember, my blood pressure was taken every 15 minutes at first, and then it was every 30 minutes and finally it was once an hour, but I still had to wear an automatic blood pressure cuff. That got uncomfortable, so I took it off my arm. Immediately the Russian nurse came in and asked, "Chris, why did you take your blood pressure cuff off?"

I was surprised, and asked her, "How did you know that?"

"We monitor everything on you, look at all these tubes you're hooked up with!"

Oh. Right. If I started moving my heart rate would change, so they could tell when I was fidgety.

She said, "We need you to lie still and just be. You're in intensive care, so let us take care of you."

But I'm Mr. Independent, Mr. Own-My-Own-Company, and I'm beginning to feel agitated because I was not able to indulge in my comfortable habits, like working until two a.m. My body was still high on sugar, but I wanted to get up, and I wanted to move around at least a little bit, which they didn't want me to do.

One of the leads came off the EKG thing I was hooked up to, and I saw how bad I was. Normally they put four or five leads on your chest for EKG, but I had leads all over my body. I'm thinking, "Oh shit, this is not good." When one of the leads popped of, the nurses monitoring me lost the signal, and the night nurse came in again and said, "No Chris! You've got to stay in bed!"

One time when I did manage to get out of bed, I had a chance to pee in the toilet. That was a big relief, because I was thinking, "Oh, my dick works! OK! Very good!" Even though I felt the pain from where that one nurse dude was shoving a catheter up there, that little sign of relief helped me start to calm down. I looked at myself in the mirror with tubes and bands and tape all over me, and I saw that I had the robe on with big armholes, and I could not help myself. I lifted my arms up like Ted Neely did in the movie *Jesus Christ Superstar*, and the theme song—"Jesus Christ, Superstar! Who in the world do you think you are?"—came into my head. I started laughing, and after that I started referring to it as my "Jesus Christ Superstar robe."

Later that night, when I felt the urge to take a shit, my stool was black. That scared me big time. If you remember the movie *Nothing in Common*, with Tom Hanks and Jackie Gleason, in the very last scene before Jackie Gleason died he had a bloody stool. Tom Hanks took him to the hospital, and Jackie Gleason died right after that. I was sitting there thinking, "Oh my God, I'm just like Jackie Gleason in that movie!"

So I got the buzzer, and the Russian nurse came in and said, "Now what?"

I whimpered to her, "Help, I just had a black stool."

She said, "Chris, sit down, let me explain this to you. That is okay because your body is healing." And she explained what the black stuff was.

Now, it didn't look like shit, and it didn't smell like shit, so when I saw it, it scared me. When you shit black it's like, "Uh-oh, now what?" That was one of those smack-yourself-up-the head, this-is-real kind of thing. So I saw black in the stool and thought, "That's my death."

The nurse said, "No, that's all the toxins. You have to get those out, so that's okay; just flush it. And stay in this bed!" After she'd explained that,

I knew that I was in the best of hands. So this time I stayed in bed. I was still very scared, very tense and alone.

Later that night, Dr. Kamath told me the hard truths that I had to face. Statistically, he practically gave me a death sentence. He was trying to scare me, I think, and I see why he might have thought I needed a smack up against the head to drive home the point of how severe my condition was, and that I had almost lost my life. His job was to not only help me to heal, but to get me to accept my new reality.

"Chris, you're a diabetic now," he finally said.

I didn't realize how long the healing process was going to be, but I made up my mind right then and there. "I haven't died yet," I thought. "I'm going to beat this." I didn't know what I was getting in to, but the only analogy I could think of at the time was rowing a boat toward a new destination; where exactly I was going, I didn't know. I didn't know what I would have to do or how I was going to pay for it. But the faith side of me heard God promising me, "I got it, Chris. Lean on me, and watch what I will do in your life."

Faith was all I had. I didn't have the government, and I didn't have income. What I had was faith, belief in myself, and my disease. Those were my three things, and I had to deal with them. I had inner turmoil, but I was not going to be a victim. What I did was embrace what my medical team was saying. I realized that I owned my body, and I was the only one who could take care of it. I had to listen.

Dr. Kamath told me a word that I hated the most—*can't*—and he said it over and over. You can't eat this anymore, Chris; you can't do these actions anymore. You have to do this, you have to eat food in five sittings, you have to take your insulin three times a day, and blah, blah, blah—and all the blah, blah, blahs were bad, bad, bad.

After the doctor left, there were only the usual three or so hospital TV channels that you could watch, and the night nurses were coming in periodically. They were all nice to me, but it was just me in there, really. After a while Momma Cille left, and it was just me and God and the sounds of the ICU—the beeping and clicking from monitors and machines, the occasional buzz of a telephone, and soft footsteps on the floor.

Most patients in the ICU were unconscious, but I was wide awake and aware of everything going on around me. I saw people coming in and leaving;

I saw entire families crying. I had to occupy my mind. So what I started to do was pray for the others around me. I was thinking, "God, this woman's crying because she's losing somebody in the room next to me. Whoever's in the room next to me, God, heal this person, heal the family." I think a death had happened. There were many people that were very upset, and I'm sitting there thinking, "I am alive, I am still able to pray for people and still able to bring them joy, so let me try to focus on this instead of myself."

The nurses wouldn't give me the details of what was going on in the bay next door to me, because they couldn't, but they did tell me it was pretty bad. So I prayed that God would have mercy on their souls, and Momma Cille, when she was there, she prayed for them too.

In between the nurses taking blood and me slowly weaning off all the sugar, I felt both vulnerable and the need to be masculine at the same time. Guys—you know, we're the alpha people who are wired to be the hunter-gatherers, as Don would say. But I realized I might as well just deal with it. So I thought of songs, I hummed, I prayed, and in between I watched the three crap channels that were on TV. I was craving Fox News and Fox Business News.

As I'm getting stuck in the middle of the night over and over with needles to monitor my blood sugar and give me insulin, it began to dawn on me that I was no longer Chris. I was now Chris the Diabetic, and I didn't like it. I tried to lean on my personality, my smile and my humor. When I was alone, I never cried, but I did feel the agony inside. I thought about Jesus' Agony in the Garden, too. Because every time they stuck me, it was a bitter reminder that was going to have to do this for the rest of my life.

Ma took a picture of me on her cell phone and emailed it to Damion. In the photo I still had the old' Chris smile—as Don would say, "Awww, there's the Chris Smile"—but when I saw the image of myself laying in ICU all puffy, I barely looked like myself. I knew I was not good. I was really, really bad off.

It's truly a miracle that I'm even here today. By the books, by every logical argument, I should be dead. I think part of what was going on is that I had gotten to the point of lowest self-esteem, where I felt so bad about myself that—well, I didn't want to die, but I accepted that I would. But I put my faith and trust in God, because He had sent me my guardian angel. If my grandmother had not been Lucille Mungo Lynch—overbearing, controlling Momma Cille—I would be dead.

5

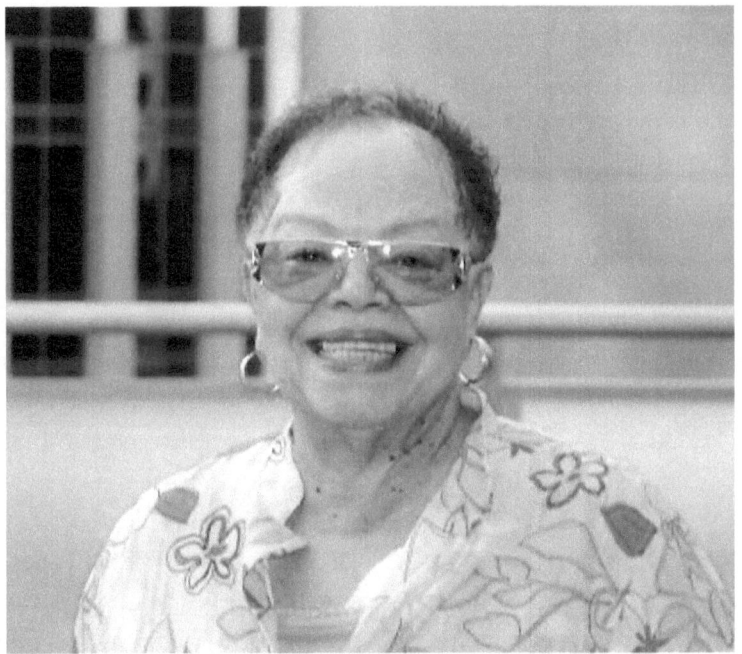

The Matriarch and the Bishop

Ma had just buried the second of her three children.

My mother Patricia was Momma Cille's oldest daughter, and Aunt Phyllis was her middle child. My Uncle Arthur, who is my cousins' Patrick and Deirdre's dad, was her baby. Aunt Phyllis died in December 2007, and ten months after Aunt Phyllis passed, I ended up in ICU.

The Monday night before I ended up in the ICU, I was so weak that my Blackberry phone slipped out of my hand into a cup of lemonade in my car, and I lost all my contact numbers that had been on it. I found out later that many people thought I had died, because I normally would talk to them a lot and hadn't called them. I didn't have my laptop, so I didn't have email. The guy who is constantly on the phone and constantly in touch with people had simply disappeared.

The next day, Wednesday, I still could not eat or drink anything. I was trying to sweet talk my way into getting something to drink from the nurses but they refused. They told me they had to get me back to a stable position before I could drink anything. I remember asking them why they couldn't just give me a few bags of fluid and let me out of there.

I became good friends with my nurses, especially when they told me they were purposefully keeping me in ICU my entire stay because I made them laugh in the midst of death. At one point, I had feces on me when I lost control of my bowels, and after wiping me up, one of the nurses had a little bottle of something that she squirted up my anus. I called it the "incontinent after spray," because it tingled like after shave. It felt pretty good, and it smelled good, so I told the nurse, "That feels good, can you leave that bottle in here?" When she asked me why, I said, "I don't know, just in case!" She burst out laughing.

I started making up this whole joke about the bags of stuff they were putting in my IV. When the nurses came to change the IV bags, I would say, "So what are we getting in that bag today? Oh, this one's filet mignon and that one's fried chicken, right?" I had to fantasize about something! When the nurse finally let me have a tiny cup of Diet Sprite, it felt like nectar from the gods going down my throat.

Late Wednesday afternoon, Tony had come in to visit me when a nurse brought in my first real food—a bowl of dark broth. They were giving me food as an experiment because my blood sugar was so high there was no record of how to treat it. I felt like I was sitting in a petri dish. The nurse encouraged me to eat all of it, and Tony was joining in, telling me to eat the broth because it was good for me. But it was so nasty, I couldn't stomach it.

Tony insisted, and I told him, "Listen, this stuff is nasty! If you think it's so great, you try it." So he swallowed a spoonful of it and almost vomited. He used to work in the food industry, but he was incredulous at how bad the stuff tasted. After I saw the look on his face, I said to him, "Yeah, not even Mikey wants to eat this!"

The nurse laughed and said, "Chris, we have to rebuild your body. If you think about it, that's industrial-strength health in that bowl."

I couldn't believe it. "Well, it tastes like canned shit!" Tony said he felt so bad for me that he wanted to go across the street to Bojangles and get me real food. But those days were over.

I wish I had a picture of my arms during that hospital stay, to document the needle pricks and bruising. I had my blood drawn constantly. At one point during the night, a respiratory therapist had to come in to take my blood, because my veins had collapsed. She had to take the blood from my artery, and that was really painful. I looked up at her and whimpered, "Hold me!" My arms started to look like I had gone to war! My medical records contain pages and pages of all the times they gave me a shot or medicine, and it just goes on and on.

But in the face of all that, the nurses said, "Oh no, he won't die! We've got him." The nurses would tell me, "Chris, we love you, but we don't want to see you back here, because that would mean you were really sick." So there was a lot of love, a lot of concern, and a lot of humor, but inside of me the fear was trying to take me. It was a battle, because I was trying to be as calm and cool as I possibly could while sitting there thinking, "Oh, my God, what am I going to do?"

I remember looking down at all tubes, leads and wires I was hooked up to and thinking, "I'm connected up to all this?" It was traumatic realizing how dependent I was on other people. I was terrified, and I didn't know how to articulate my fear. I was driven to be positive, calm, and happy with the people there, but inside, I was lonely. I wanted to cry; I wanted to emote from the trauma.. I wished that I had someone to share my innermost thoughts. I had lots of people in my life, but no girlfriend or wife. What I wanted to say to the nurse was, "I really want someone to hold me and help me through this."

Momma Cille would tell me stories, like about how the day Martin Luther King died in 1968 was also my birthday, April 4. Damion's birthday is April 5, so sometimes we would have a collective birthday celebration, usually on my birthday. But my memories of Momma Cille were as my mother.

My faith came from Momma Cille; she modeled my faith. That's why I get a feeling of excitement when it's Catholic Schools week, because she made sure that all of us went to Catholic schools, and I had simply loved the times I had in those schools. Now just for the record, it's not that she though public schools were bad. But she loved Catholicism, and my belief in the traditional Church came from her belief.

She was not a materialistic person, but she did like to dream big. I remember once when I bought her a big bunch of flowers she said, "Chris, that's so sweet! But why don't you put that money into a Lotto ticket?" That was Momma Cille. She was always appreciative if you did anything for her; she'd go on and on about it, to fully express her gratitude. If you gave her anything at Christmas: "Oh, this is so nice!" she'd say. Then she'd go on to say, "And such pretty wrapping paper!" Deirdre, Patrick and all of us would laugh every Christmas, because Ma would take so much time opening her presents. "I don't want to mess up the pretty bows," she'd say. Afterward she'd sit there and call all of her friends to report on what she had gotten.

Ma loved fancy things, so I'd bring her the luxury lifestyle magazine *Robb Report.* I'd tell her, "Ma, even though we can't afford expensive things, we can at least dream about them." She loved to look through that magazine. She'd say, "Oh boy, who makes Maserati, Chris?"

"Um, Ma, Maserati," I'd laugh.

"Is that a nice car?"

"Yeah, Ma, it's pretty nice."

"Oh, yeah!" she'd nod. "I think I want one of those."

Now if somebody did something she didn't approve of, she'd say, "I'm going to call them and give them a piece of my mind!" She'd express her feelings. But then she'd say, "No, I don't want to waste a cent on them, they're one of God's children." If she knew you were Catholic, you could do no wrong in her eyes. The innocence of a child, a simple trust in God, was what her faith was like.

Her daily prayer regimen was to wake up, say her rosary, and say the divine chaplet—officially the Chaplet of Divine Mercy. It consists of the Our Father, the Hail Mary, and the Apostle's Creed. Ma loved Mother Angelica and Chris Matthews and that's she watched on TV—CNN and EWTN, which is the global Catholic television network. She was always

Prayer Central, really. Momma Cille *believed*. She was the personification of unshakeable faith in Jesus Christ; that's the best way that I can articulate it, and she lived her faith with her actions. She carried her cross and she carried her faith with her no matter where she was.

The first time I truly understood Ma's connection to God was when I experienced my own. I clearly remember during my confirmation in eighth grade. When Bishop Michael Begley put the chrism on my forehead. I felt the true presence of the Holy Spirit. First Communion was not a big deal for me, even though it probably should have been since it was when I first experienced the Eucharist. At my confirmation, I felt for the first time God's presence in my life. It was April of 1980, the March or April right before Pentecost.

The second moment when I felt my faith increase—and this is going to sound crazy—was February 1, 1984, the night of my very first Van Halen concert. In my head as a child, I would hear these rock 'n' roll sounds and tones, and that internal music was a fuel for my faith. So when I say that I had a religious experience at a Van Halen concert, let me tell you what I mean.

I remember it was a *cold* day, and I was in my last year of high school. I was so excited; I remember I stood outside the Charlotte Coliseum with Charlotte Catholic friends wearing my Members Only jacket, and we were all screaming and carrying on 'til we got inside. The lights went out, and then Van Halen came on the stage, and Eddie Van Halen played, note for note, the tones I had been hearing in my head. He *reproduced* them on the stage. It was the weirdest thing in the world. I felt like God used Eddie to talk personally to me and say, "I'm here, too—in the music."

From that moment forward, Van Halen's music was another source of spiritual fuel for me, a pure form of energy that powered my life. I felt God's presence in Eddie's music. I can promise you that he didn't know he was doing it, but that first moment was pure religiosity, if that's even a word. Or, as Don King said in the documentary about himself, he had an "epiphanous experience of pure religiosity." I had a replication of my confirmation experience, and I think God was saying, "Chris, here's the creative ability that you have inside you, and I gave it to this person (Eddie) too."

I was weepy, I was shaking; it was as if that music flipped my switches *on*. I realize that moment with me and the Van Halen concert is probably hard for people to fully understand, but it's true. I think that's part of the reason why, when crazy happens, a calmness just comes over me to deal with whatever is facing me, because I hear music.

When I was laying on the gurney in the emergency room, and the doctor was telling me, "Mr. Lynch, I don't know if you even know this, but you're dying," I was like, "Okay, well, no cross, no crown, I guess I deserve this." But God's mercy was with me, because in the back of my mind, I was saying, "God, I'm a person who loves You so much, and I want to be who you created me to be, a happy human being so I can help other people." I think the intervention of Mother Teresa, who Bishop Curlin called on to help me, and the prayers of Bishop Curlin, along with Blanche and Momma Cille, were what saved me. I would be dead today, if God had not used those individuals to pray on my behalf.

Momma Cille and Bishop William G. Curlin had been good friends since 1994, when he had succeeded Bishop John Donoghue. The joke in the family was that Bishop Curlin was our family priest, because if any tragedy happened, any situation, he'd always show up. He'd bring Ma communion if she couldn't get out to mass, and when he'd make his run to the hospital, he'd always stop by to visit Ma at her home. They had a very good relationship. I wasn't going to mass at the time, so I said to Ma, "You've got to call Bishop Curlin. Please get him over here." I needed to be anointed—the sacrament that some call the last rites.

Bishop Curlin has what I call spiritual confidence—almost to the brink of spiritual arrogance—but in a good way. For example, he always takes a group to Lourdes—if not once a year, it's twice a year—because when he had cancer and other illnesses, he was healed there at the grotto. He's a very loving, jovial person, and he pretty much smiles all the time.

Before I was discharged from the hospital Friday morning, Bishop Curlin came to see me that Wednesday. Momma Cille was in the room with me, and so was Blanche. This was during the day in the early afternoon between one and three. The nurse started to come in and saw that Bishop Curlin was there, so she started to leave the room.

I called out to her, "Oh no, come on in, this is Catholic—this is cool!" But she said, "No, I'll give you guys some privacy."

I remember when he came in, I could feel the warmth and grace of God fill the entire room. When he administered the Anointing of the Sick to me, I felt very Catholic then, if that makes any sense. The only two sacraments I hadn't received were Holy Orders and Anointing of the Sick, and when he gave me that sacrament that was number six of seven. I remember thinking, "Wow, I'm getting the sixth sacrament—this is awesome!" Of course, most people would probably not be thrilled at that, because it's obviously a very serious moment. Yet Bishop Curlin was very calming and loving towards me. Just Jesus-filled, asking for my healing.

I have never forgotten what the Bishop said to me then. He sat by the bed and said, "Chris I'm going to give you this sacrament, and then I'm going home, and I'm going to say a mass especially for you. I know you're going to heal, because my stuff works."

At that moment, I felt like God gave me Himself through Bishop Curlin to say, "Chris, now you are going to earn Me." Meaning, I'm going to feel the fullness of God's presence in my life. It passed to me through Bishop Curlin.

I remember Don, whom I call the Eternal Protestant because he almost *wants* to be Catholic, because he seems to admire the traditions so much but for some reason won't go there, was very impressed. He said to people afterwards, "Christopher had the Bishop Emeritus of the Diocese of Charlotte come in and give him Extreme Unction[4]!" You'd have to hear him say that in his genteel Southern gentleman voice. The moment Bishop Curlin put the cross on my forehead with blessed oil was the beginning of my journey.

I put my faith and trust in Bishop Curlin's words, and felt a child-like acceptance of belief. I clung to his words: "My stuff works." This situation was almost identical to my confirmation and Van Halen experiences. I'm there in the most vulnerable of vulnerable positions, lying in the bed with tubes, needles, and that stupid blood pressure cuff that until this day I

---

4 "Extreme Unction" was a western, technical term for this Roman Catholic Rite, used after the Council of Trent until 1972, when the Constitution of the Liturgy declared that "anointing" of the sick was a more fitting term. The term "extreme unction" is rarely used today.

can still feel squeezing my arm. But this fell away in that moment when Bishop Curlin came in and a new journey began that put me on the path and led me where I am today. The peace that I feel at every Sunday mass has grown in me from that moment back in October 2008.

Until Bishop Curlin came in to the ICU, I was in denial. My illness and everything that was happening to me felt like a bad dream, and I couldn't get past the pain and fear, so I just pushed it away. But after the Sacrament, I was given the grace and the faith to deal with it.

I heard everything the doctors and nurses were saying, and I understood all the statistics they cited, such as, 65 percent of deaths in people with diabetes are due to heart disease and stroke. You know, most medical people are all about facts—they're not dealing with the spiritual, and it's all about telling you what the medical reports say—blah, blah, blah. But what I *knew* was that Bishop Curlin was saying "my stuff works;" that I *would* be healed. So that was my lubrication, shall we say, the thing that powered my path to follow. He went home to what I call Our Lady of Bishop Curlin's House, his own private chapel, and said mass there for me, and I could feel the grace from that. The metaphysical and spiritual part of my experience, I could not discuss with my medical team at the hospital, but Bishop Curlin gave me that inoculation from God, and it gave me the strength to face the battle that was ahead of me.

I truly started feeling better as soon as Bishop Curlin put the oil on my forehead. I felt the God injection! The only way I could describe the rock-bottom feeling I had before that was imagining a wet, oily, nasty, soot-filled hole, and I was wallowing in the middle of it. But when I looked up, there was light.

On Thursday I was told I was out of danger.

Ashleigh Thore was a nutritionist at CMC-Pineville who gave me my continuing diabetes education. Ashleigh visited that Thursday, and she was the person that brought it all together for Chris the Diabetic. She explained to me how to give myself insulin shots, in what are called preferred sites, and that they were going to wean me off the IV and encourage me to give myself the shots.

I remember Ashleigh vividly, because I was trying to get a little bit of sleep. Being pricked and prodded the whole time was wearing me out. Every time they came in and tested something or gave me another shot, it woke me up. When Ashleigh came in and said, "Hi," I actually jumped in my skin, because she startled me.

I told her, "Ashleigh, you are the one I've been looking forward to talking to, because I need the dumbass version of nutrition. I need to take Dumbass Nutrition 101."

She said, "Chris, it's not that difficult, I'll help you." I shared with her that I was intimidated about going to the grocery store and having to read all the labels, count calories, and worrying about the foods I could eat.

I told her, "I feel like I'm swimming in the deep end of the pool now, and if I don't swim right I'll drown. I have to live, and I want to live, and I really need your help."

She was the first person who helped me to understand that nutrition is a way of life, not a diet. I had heard people often say that forming a new habit can take three to four weeks, but if you stick with it that long it will become habitual.

Another nurse taught me how to test my blood sugar, and she patiently answered every question I had. She and Ashleigh told me that we could dive into nutrition and living with diabetes as much as I wanted. They explained to me what hyperglycemia and hypoglycemia were, and the signs and symptoms of each.

Ashleigh explained that hypoglycemia could give me the shakes, and that the shakes would indicate that I was extremely hungry and extremely weak. At all cost, I wanted to avoid that. Becoming that hungry was a result of my body processing all the sugar I had available in my body for energy, and the hunger was almost saying, "More, more!" Because of the possibility of hypoglycemia, I needed to have on standby a sugar-induced food, such as three or four pieces of hard candy or a sweet drink, like orange juice. But they also explained that I needed to stay away from juice except for when I'm hypoglycemic, because juice would dump too much sugar into my bloodstream.

The other thing I had to completely understand was going the other way into hyperglycemia. I learned that hyperglycemia gives one a fast heart rate, irritability, and listlessness, and that if I was hypoglycemic in the morning, it meant my body had exhausted its insulin reserves.

If it had not sunk in by now, the detailed healthcare regimen I had to follow from now on did. I counted up what I had to do, and I realized

I was going to have to stick myself with a needle eight times a day: three shots of insulin, and five times to check my blood sugar.

I learned there were crucial times during the day in which I needed to check my blood sugar. Of course the most important time was when I woke up in the morning, so I knew what my body had done during the night. Ashleigh said that because I was in such a severe situation, I needed to check my blood sugar again before noon, once in the mid-afternoon, in the evening before dinner, and just before I went to bed. Checking five times a day would remind me to eat five times a day, too; smaller meals that would help me maintain a good balance.

She said if I got into an extreme state—hypo- or hyperglycemic—I would have to check my sugar. I thought to myself, "Man, I'm going to *really* be mad at myself if I have to check my sugar six or more times a day because I got out of balance." So I started telling myself that I was going to stick to my regimen.

I don't have any words to explain the anxiety and anger that hit me when I realized how many times I would be staring down a needle. I used to get anxious three months before going to the doctor for a physical. Even though Ashleigh told me that all of this would become routine, I simply could not accept that I would have to stick myself eight times every day for what was looking like the rest of my life.

I have to tell you that even now, I hate the feeling of checking my sugar, but I anticipate seeing my number, because today, I'm chasing the number. Because I know the numbers to look for, I don't have as much anxiety about it anymore. But sitting in ICU learning how to use a blood sugar meter was definitely one of my lower points. I had to accept that when I left the hospital, I still was never going to be completely well.

Because I'm an electronic geek, I dug that my meter had a digital display, and I wanted to learn everything about how it reads your sugar from a tiny bit of blood. There was also an art to getting the finger prick right so I didn't end up having to stick myself over and over to get a reading. Everyone has something that bothers more than anything else, like the sound of scrapes on a chalkboard, or the click of a fork against the teeth. Well, I have two. One of those is listening to people who chew gum openly, with that smacking, wet breathing sound. That drives me insane. The other one is pricking my finger and pushing the blood out for my meter reading.

In the hospital, Ashleigh explained what a lancet was, and they showed me how to use an old school insulin reading tool, where I had to pick up a lancet, take the plastic cap off it, and stare down a big, stabbing thing. I then had to put the lancet in its little device, cock it, basically, almost like a gun, and then fire it into my finger.

I'm telling you, staring down that damned thing as well as the bigger needle that I had to use three times a day to give myself insulin shots took more courage than I ever thought it would. I call it the "getting stuck" anxiety. I would tense up, anticipating the pain, and even though I knew I would survive it, it seemed my whole body would tighten up. Every time, I wanted someone to hold me and say, "It's OK, Chris. It's OK." Because it sucked.

The other issue I had is using alcohol. I simply can't stand the smell of isopropyl alcohol. It reminds me of being a kid and being seen at the Nalle Clinic, and watching my grandfather Arthur stick himself. What I did instead was just wash my hands and dry them roughly so there was no water conducting on my skin that would repel the blood.

With insulin, I had to learn to alternate sites, which I also hated. They taught me to stick myself in my abdomen, but I couldn't bear the thought of the pain of doing that on a regular basis, whether it was on my right side or my left. I tried to stick my abdomen once when I was back home, but I was shaking so bad that I dropped the needle. And then I had the Howard Hughes fear. I had heard that when he was found dead, Hughes had a bunch of needles stuck into his arms. I don't know why that knowledge stuck in my mind, but I remember watching a "20/20" episode years ago where they were showing an image of Howard Hughes taking needles.

I couldn't do arm because the arms are not preferred sites for insulin, so I settled on sticking myself in my legs, as they were the point of least resistance; I could at least stand to stick myself without shaking like a baby. So I learned to stick my left leg, and then my right leg, alternating each time.

I laughed and joked with the nurses during my diabetic training. When they asked me if I was ready to stick myself from now on, I begged off, knowing they would take pity on me. Part of me was afraid to mess up in front of them, but I also felt this was something I was going to have to do alone.

I had my faith, and my faith renewed me, even though I knew I was never going to be happy about being a diabetic. I trusted in God, but I wasn't sure I trusted myself. I really wanted to break out of my old patterns. God had saved me, but was my new life going to end up being like my last?

6

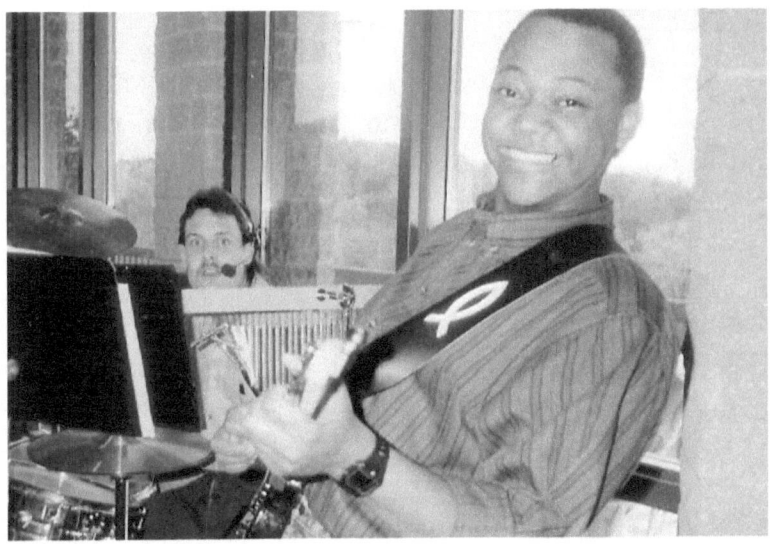

Red flags

I met my wife at church.

Sister Antoinette at Charlotte Catholic did retreats in the mountains for a lot of kids during the 80s, and before my high school graduation I participated in one. There were kids there from lots of different parishes throughout the Charlotte diocese.

When I was working at General Medical in the early 90s, I was back up in that area visiting and went to mass on Sunday. Before mass began, I heard a female voice say, "Chris?" When I turned toward the voice, I was re-acquainted with a girl I had met on that retreat named Helen.

Helen had just graduated from college and was moving to a town close to me to teach in a school there. I thought, "That will be cool, we can be good friends." I gave her my number and suggested we get together, and we started meeting at mass and going out after.

For me at that time, my spiritual zest had begun to fade. Michael W. Smith has a song called "Going Through the Motions," and that song speaks to me because that's what I felt I was doing. I wanted to have an even deeper faith, but I was afraid to go further. I was not in the most connected point of my spirituality yet, but I was always trying to put my faith into the middle of my life. I thought if I attended mass regularly, I'd be doing something good and wholesome, and people would like me for that. Being at church was what people normally saw me doing, so I thought I might as well stay there.

We started going out on dates and then, kind of quickly, I became the guy that hung out with Helen. She was attractive, but she was the quintessential virgin. She had no dating experience at all.

I had a hard time connecting with her. For weeks on end I tried desperately just to kiss her, but Helen would put up huge red flags around herself. When I think back to it now, she was probably trying to tell me to get the hell away from her. She seemed to be in love with my personality, though—the extroverted, always happy Chris. I think she wanted to make me happy, and she did care for me.

I also saw Helen as something of a challenge. I was convinced I could make her happy and that we could build a life together. I got to know her parents and her brother, and they all liked me and seemed happy about a match between us. But Helen was uncomfortable with being a bi-racial couple, and about the prospect of having sex.

Being with a white woman never bothered me. I was never embarrassed or angry even if people stared. I just did not care what others thought about me, frankly. I was determined to be with Helen, despite the early signs she displayed that should have told me she did not want a permanent relationship. Yet, she never actually pushed me away. At this time there were other beautiful women making passes at me at the time, from work and other places, but I didn't pay any attention to them because I was concentrating on getting that crown—a Catholic, Christian marriage— which meant I had to struggle.

It was a simple reality to me. I had to struggle in order to be happy because the cross—struggle, suffering, and all that bullshit—was the only way to get what I wanted. Helen insisted on remaining a virgin until we got married, and I accepted that. I thought I could be a good guy and accept the temporary chastity. But I felt like I was becoming her doormat.

Momma Cille was supportive of our relationship, and sometimes I think I wanted the attention that marriage would give me with her, instead of wanting to be married because I loved Helen. Damion was doing well and getting a lot of attention, and I was feeling, again, left out. I felt like I always had to run up the hill four times faster than other people to get noticed in my family.

I was determined to get this girl, because I thought if we got married, and it's all Catholic and sacramental and all of that, I'd be responsible. Finally! I'll be responsible in someone's eyes! But inside, I never had that little nervous feeling in my stomach that told me, "Wow, she really cares for me."

I didn't have a college degree, and that was uncomfortable for Helen because she had a degree in education and her parents were academics. Her Mom and Dad never condemned me for it, but they'd say things like, "Chris, maybe it would be good for you to go back one day and get your degree." But Helen kept bringing up the fact that I didn't have a degree, and bragging to me about the school she attended.

She kept up the pressure by talking about my wasted potential and how I couldn't be somebody without a degree. So I went back to the Abbey to finish my B.A.

I was able to get back into the theology program. I received credit for all the liturgical experience I had gained, and only had to take a few more classes to graduate. I'm glad I did it, because I gained a sense of completion. But what I really loved was selling technology. When I moved to my next job, my raw selling skills were the most important thing.

We dated about two years before I asked her to marry me. It was my Mom's birthday, September 16, so it was a special night for me. When most women get an engagement ring, they never stop talking about it. Helen, however, never said a thing about the ring I put on her finger. She never showed it to her girlfriends or anything. It was like you had to pull it out of her. This should have been a huge red flag!

Couples who marry in the Roman Catholic Church must complete pre-marriage counseling under the guidance of a priest. You fill out a questionnaire before you go, and one of the first things you do is discuss the answers on the questionnaires. When Helen and I started counseling, the priest said to us, "Chris and Helen, there's a whole lot of stuff here that we have to get through, because you guys are not on the same page."

We went through six or seven counseling sessions, where most people have about two. In the end, I don't think the priest felt completely OK about our marrying, but he saw no impediment to the Sacrament, so he gave us the thumbs up. But those sessions should have been an even bigger red flag.

Instead of sitting down and talking with her, saying, "You know Helen, this is a mistake," I felt that we were already on the path now, and we had gone too far to stop. We've told people, we've scheduled time, we've got everything out there; we couldn't go backwards. Rather than stopping when I had the chance, I once again chose that path of least resistance.

I think more people talked about the fact that we were making a mistake than I realized. I know people in our families did, but no one came to me and said, "Chris, stop. Don't do this." Don was the only one that tried, but I was defensive about it, which may have been why my family did not try to intervene. I know now that the struggle and the pain was giving me life, instead of the joy and faith I really needed. Pain was what I was running on.

Close to the end of our relationship when we were in couples therapy, Helen admitted to me that she went into our marriage thinking, "Chris is a nice guy. Maybe what I'll do is get into the middle of it, and it will all get better down the road." But we would soon learn that marriage was only going to make us more distant from one another.

Don was my best man. Helen was walking down the aisle to Pachelbel's Canon, and as she approached us, Don leaned over to me and said, "Chris! You don't have to do this. Run!" He was not saying it to be funny, either. He had seen the look on Helen's face that I did. She looked like that church was the last place she wanted to be in.

I looked back at Don as if to say, "Huh? No, I'm fine." But inside I was miserable. I knew I was getting ready to eat a bowl of soup that had already gone stone cold.

Being married to Helen never felt right, even from the very first. I remember when we were riding down the mountain to go on our honeymoon, I told myself, "Oh man, I really did it!" I had already lost my virginity, but Helen had never had sex with anybody. I was proud that I had waited for her. I even remember taking a picture of someone who asked me, "Hey, Chris, are you happy?" and responding, "Yeah, I'm going to get laid!" I thought I had been this good guy, and everything would be great from then on. Was I ever up for an awakening.

A friend of Helen's gave us a "honeymoon night kit" that I thought was a cool gift. Her friend was a highly sensual person, and I couldn't help wondering why Helen was not more sensual, too. Her friend was the kind of person that when she'd hug you, you'd feel the need to take a couple of steps back because it felt a little *too* good. Now I was never the cheating type, but I would feel bad for even thinking about such a thing when I was with Helen.

On that first night of married life, Helen was petrified of having sex, so I promised to wait until the next night. One night turned into a week, and that week turned into a month. Then Helen said, "Well you know Chris, we're going to be moving to Maryland. Why don't we just wait until then, and I promise I'll do better." I said to her, "I am here for you, and I trust you. I know you wouldn't let me down."

But I remembered a joke she made before we got married, that maybe wasn't a joke. She had told me that a friend of hers had gotten married recently, and that she thought it was cool that they played poker the night of the honeymoon and didn't have sex for a few days. That was an indication right there that we were not going to make it. Nevertheless, I could not face that fear—the fear that I had failed yet again.

Two weeks after we were married we moved to Maryland so I could begin my new job at a major bank. I was in a branch management trainee program, and Helen eventually found a teaching job as an elementary teacher at a nearby school. Everyday life set in.

The month turned into six months, and Helen somehow managed to keep putting me off. Every time I'd try to make an advancement in that department, she would make me feel bad for asking her questions to find out what I was doing wrong. I would say, "Helen, you're my wife and I love you." But she would say, "Chris, all you ever think about is sex."

I was embarrassed to talk about this issue with anyone else. One of my teammates at the bank was a typical DC native—butt-ass blunt. I love people that are like that, because with them you never have to mince words, and you know where you stand. She called the trainees her knuckleheads. She'd been married and had two kids.

One day she said to me, "Chris, you look tense."

I shrugged it off and said something about work making me tired.

She said, "You know what you need to do? You need to go home, throw your wife on the bed and fuck her brains out."

I laughed, but not because I thought that was funny. I was actually laughing because she had no idea what I was going home to face! During the entirety of our marriage, we did not have sex. Not once.

The anguish I was feeling was unbearable. I tried everything to make our relationship work. Helen's brother visited us at the house in Maryland, and he and I got along great. To this day I still can't quite define what caused that rejection, and I don't know what her perspective on it was. Helen said she didn't know why she could not face having sex.

Her Mom and Dad were devastated when they found out about it. Her Mom asked once, "Hey, when are we going to see some kids?"

I said to her, "We have to have sex before we have kids."

"Oh no, you haven't had sex yet?" she said. I had to tell her again. "No, we have not had sex." They were completely baffled.

I loved Helen's parents and her brother Johnny. He and I bonded; Johnny was like Mike in my life at that time. Mike was never replaced, but Johnny and I had the same sense of camaraderie and humor and we were both musicians. He's a guitar player, and very accomplished, much more so than me. He was into very complicated guitar licks, and he loved bands like Toto. He could really emulate a lot of lead guitar playing. I was a very good rhythm guitar player, but he was the lead guitar player that I struggled to be. I never felt intimidated by him, though, because we could always have a meeting of the minds.

One memory I have illustrates the relationship I had with Johnny and Helen when we were all together. Helen had this thing where she would get upset if she thought I said anything remotely sexual, because that meant I was criticizing her.

I said to Johnny, "Hey man, let's play the lick game." We'd sit there and listen to music and go back and forth, saying, "Tell me, what's your best guitar lick?"

Helen got completely upset. She said something like, "Don't use that lingo, it's gross!" Anything I said, she assumed it was something sexual.

I said, "No, I'm talking about guitar licks!" I was so frustrated. I wanted to say, "Look, you're my wife and I can't have sex with you! At least let me find some pleasure!" I never actually said that, but I was just swimming in hate and pain.

Helen's suggestion that I might be trying to send her passive-aggressive sexual signs was the worst, because I'm pretty direct about stuff. Sometimes I hear women say, "My man doesn't pay attention to me." They would not be able to say that about me. I did all the things you're supposed to do. It didn't get me anywhere, though. I tried every way I could think about. Inside, I told myself, "I'm not letting this one go; hell no. I'm going to get this girl at any cost."

At work I had no problem making close friends with women. They used to say things like, "I wish you weren't taken, Chris." But I could not respond to that because I was on a mission. I had to go swimming in the right or left side of the Red Sea, when I could have been walking on the parted land. By choice. Even though with Helen, giving her any affection at all was like trying to get a Q-tip through a pinhead.

I thought I was in love with her. I didn't know what love was, because I understand now you have to have self-love before you can give love. I think what I had was definitely infatuation, but I never was in love with her. I realized that later, when I got into my next relationship, because I truly was in love with that woman, who later moved with me into the big Charlotte house. But when I think back on my life with Helen, like in my lonely moments, I have no memories of good times when we were together. It was the worst pain I'd been through in my life, because it was as if I had to deal with a living death. The fact is, Helen didn't trust me. With the controlling women in my life, trust was, I believe, really the issue. And Helen was the epitome of a controlling woman.

It was always her way or the highway. She would be very snippy with me, and she'd insist on refraining from public affection. Now I'm a very affectionate, loving, hugging kind of person, but Helen wouldn't even allow me to hold her hand in public.

I started giving her these little jabs, as if to fight back. I knew the way to get to her was her vanity, because she was always about making herself look good. I remember one time she pissed me off about one thing or another, and I said, "You know, I've seen you better," and walked out of the room. She immediately changed her outfit. I knew just how to flip that switch in her. It was wrong, because I was just measuring tit for tat, you know. But that celibate pain—we were together four years! To refuse to have sex with me was the ultimate form of rejection.

She'd say things like, "Hey, how you doing today?" as if we were strangers passing by. I wanted her to at least treat me like a human being, but I seemed to be an entity to Helen; I was a thing.

Helen didn't seem to know how to relate or how to love, perhaps because she did not love herself. I was in my own pool of mess, too, because by not loving myself, I didn't know how to receive love from anyone else. My friend Pam used to ask me, "Why can't you find somebody that gives you back as much as you give?" But when she'd say that, I didn't understand what she meant. I knew that she was talking about the possibility of real happiness, but I never could force myself to articulate my pain or say that I was not happy. I couldn't let myself feel good; I had to struggle.

I continued to do well at work, but my numbness continued to build. I remember one time when I was in a meeting, I twisted my neck to stretch it, and it made this loud cracking sound. One of my work buddies said to me, "Dude, are you alright?"

I shrugged it off. "No man, I'm fine. I'm just tired." But inside I wanted to just scream. I had this tight, tense feeling inside, like a big knot. My refuge, of course, was food. With Helen, I basically ate trash. I gained about 25 pounds, and I felt *round*. I knew I was unhealthy, but I could not stop. When I thought about it, I'd tell myself I had to find some kind of peace. I'm married, I can't have sex, and I don't have my Mom—I could have written a really good blues song! The chorus would be, "Junk food, TV and pain." Overeating was my escape.

I still cannot believe that I allowed myself to go as far as I did with that situation, because I was dying on the inside.

During the week we were isolated from each other because Helen was a workaholic. This is not necessarily a bad thing, but on Sunday through Thursday, she worked like a dog. As a teacher, she was grading tests when she got home and preparing her lessons. But every day wasn't a bad day. We laughed occasionally about things, and we had jokes we would tell. Saturdays were the days that we would go on little field trips.

One of the things that I appreciated about Helen is she loved to go to parks, and always seemed happiest when she was outside. Her brother always came with us, so it was the three amigos off on our little adventures. We went to Civil War battlegrounds and other places around Columbia and D.C.

Johnny used to ask, "Helen, don't you want to spend some time alone with Chris?"

She would shake her head. "No, no, we're married, we have time together every day. We are fine."

I was grateful for Johnny's company, but in many ways Helen and I were two opposites.

I love the joke that Chris Rock tells. If you're two crackheads, you'll be together forever. If one is a church-going person and the other one uses meth, it's just a matter of time before you break up. I remember feeling that way with Helen because I didn't like hiking and sightseeing that much. I don't like walking around in the heat and that kind of thing, but she was really getting off on it. That was *her* escape. I thought if I could be the good husband and give her what she wants, she would reciprocate and I would get something from her happiness, but it did not work that way.

All the same, I never thought about doing the things I used to do that made *me* happy—playing guitar and messing around with electronics. We did a few things together and the rest of the time we tried to escape from each other. My escape was watching television and listening to music with headphones; she hated when I would wear headphones. It was just like living at 609 as a kid—escaping into music. During that time, all the other things that had brought me happiness died away. I barely knew I was missing them until I met my therapist, Meg. She asked me what my hobbies were, and I had actually forgotten. I told her, "I'm boring, I can't think of anything." I had somehow become lifeless. Damion told me later that I always looked like I had a small turd under my nose when Helen was around.

One week Helen and I went to Rhode Island on a vacation. Johnny had gone somewhere alone, and I got the courage to finally try to talk about what was wrong and to get us to stop doing this to each other.

I said, "This isn't working, and we have to fix it."

She had her mind on going back to North Carolina. She talked about how she missed it . Helen was very intimidated by D.C. and the surroundings—the traffic, the Metro, and all the activity of Washington. I got off on it, but she always felt like she belonged back in North Carolina.

I insisted that we deal with things now instead of waiting, and if she wanted to go back to North Carolina, she should go. I said, "We need to make this public and start dealing with officially breaking up." As soon as we got back from the trip, we started formulating a plan. We had to live with each other for another six months until her job situation was set.

We didn't own very much, so it was very simple to break up our home. When she finished her school session that June, she moved out. She left a note, but it wasn't a "Dear John" letter; it was more of a "Goodbye, John" letter. In it she told me, "Chris, you'll find the right woman." She said she felt bad, because I was so good to her; it was her *mea culpa*. Her wedding ring was sitting on top of the letter.

We had to go through one year of separation before our divorce was final. The papers came to me on December 24. I thought they were the best Christmas present ever. I told myself I was happier then. But that was when the pain truly started to erupt. I began to feel like I was coming apart.

I remember sitting in my apartment many a night crying, feeling hurt and not knowing to do with my pain. That's why I went to therapy. It turned out to be an amazing experience. Meg was my therapist, and I started to release that huge knot of stress I had. She helped me to get through that period, and gave me permission to be myself.

Two years later, on New Year's Eve, 1999, I was doing what I usually do on New Year's Eve —sit and reflect on the year so I can start the year off on a good note. I cranked up Prince's "1999," and I said to myself, "I'm going to party; I'm going to really live life." My marriage had been annulled, and being in D.C., alone and growing, felt right. I was at the right place, I was clicking and grooving with my career, and everything was moving in the right direction.

7

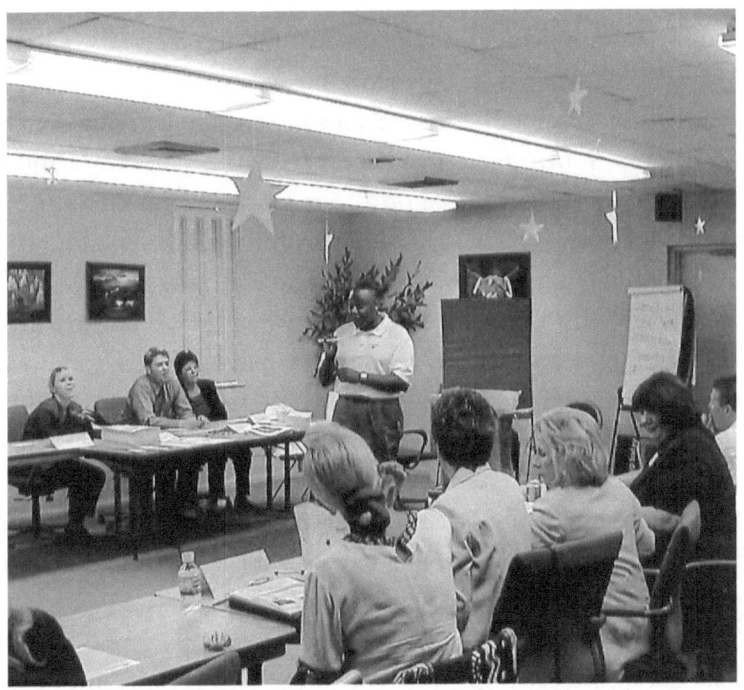

Wet Doughnuts

I had begun to feel like wet doughnuts;
so heavy I couldn't lift my head up.

After I finished the management training program at the bank, I went into training and business development, which gave me a taste of travel. I was alone with my personal problems, but I was mobile. I was traveling all over D.C. and Maryland, and the traveling helped me because I wasn't faced with myself all the time. I got a little taste of freedom. Going to many different places without having to check in with someone felt good.

I remember doing a lot of life auditing. I'd been through a hard relationship, and when I thought back, I realized I had been in some kind of steady relationship with another woman for over 12 years. After I left the Abbey, I had wanted to experience life as a young person, but I had jumped right in to several serious relationships without giving myself any time to breathe. When you're an adult everything is about responsibilities; insurance and mortgages, and more of the same. I had been dealing with all that when I really wanted to just have my fun period—you know, work, go out, have fun, go to bed, wake up, and do it all over again.

I felt weighted, and troubled. I was fine when I was busy working with people, traveling, training, and teaching people how to sell. But when I came home to my empty apartment by myself, this heaviness would push me down. Pain and happiness were synonymous for me. I felt separated from other people, as if I had to stay bound up in misery to get to where I wanted to go. I remember that people would hug me and I would tense up, because I wouldn't allow myself to bathe in the love that every human is due. I chose pain, instead of letting other people in.

Still, as bad as things were with my marriage, I'll never blame Helen for that misery, because when I had opportunities to be happy, I chose to stay in pain because that was familiar to me.

For the bank, I went around to different branches of the business. I became a go-to-guy. When there were any profit issues, I was the guy they would call to rally the troops and get tactical around how to grow the business. I made the bank a load of money; I mean millions of millions of dollars based on my selling tactics.

My tactics are all about asking the customer what they need, and tying banking products to their needs and pains, instead of trying to force fit customers with the bank's products. Many of our finance salespeople operated in a way that was overtly coercive, whereas I was more conversational. I'd talk to people about what was going in their lives and businesses, and ask a lot of questions. I would use tactics that felt natural to me, and I tried to train our people to listen and be themselves, so customers would trust them.

I tried to make it real for people, and I wasn't bullshitting with anyone. I was just the dude that would get it done. I would be myself—making jokes, talking about music and concerts and things that got me—and my potential customers— jazzed up. When I would go into meetings I would be called over all the time by one person or another: "Hey, Chris, sit over here with me!" I was Mr. Happy Guy, Mr. "Hey, how are you doing?"

That said, I refused to drink the company kool-aid. No matter what my title was, I never changed my way of operating or how. The bank wanted me to change, to grown into a senior management role at some point in time, but I refused to do it, so eventually I got locked out of the rat race for the big money jobs. Which was fine with me, really. I went to the credit card division, and I blossomed there. I did hundreds of projects that involved millions of dollars of revenue generation, and the work grew me; it stretched me. And I was rewarded for it.

In spite of my success at work, I didn't realize how crippling Helen's rejection was to me emotionally and physically. If I was with a woman and wanted to ejaculate, I couldn't. My pipes were fine, but my mind was not right. I think it is easier to break a limb than to heal your brain. Emotions take much longer to heal. I remember wishing that there was some kind of over-the-counter drug I could take to help with this pain. I hated the fact that every time I tried to make an advance into a good relationship, I couldn't.

One day after my marriage ended, a friend of mine talked to his priest about my situation with Helen. After hearing about my celibate marriage, he asked my friend, "Why didn't Chris kick some tires before he got married?"

Now, by using the phrase "kick the tires," I don't think the priest meant to convey to me his disbelief that we had not had sex before our marriage. I knew this priest very well, and he was not one to influence a Catholic man to act against doctrine. But I was not rational at the time; I was too mad. So hearing about this remark floored me.

I had always been the kid that, when Father said, "Do," or "Do not," I did, or didn't do. The Catholic Church was a part of our lives, and following doctrine was what we did. I heard a priest giving me permission to have sex before I got married, and it made me feel naïve and stupid. I thought, if a priest is telling me to fool around and try women out before I propose to them, and I'm stupid enough to think I had to be a good person, then fuck Catholicism.

What I mean by that is, I felt pure angst, and hate, for the institution. I never turned my back on God, or the Eucharist. But the Catholic Church and everything in it—priests, celibacy, all of that stuff to me became anathema. My misunderstanding affected me for a long time, and I stopped going to mass.

Almost overnight I felt hate, anger and pain boiling in me like lava. No one could answer my questions about what had happened between Helen and me, or why, and I heard a priest of the Catholic Church saying to me, you should have tried to have sex with her before you got married. But when you go to mass, the message is, "Oh, no! Don't even think about that!"

As I looked back on all my experiences, and everything I missed out on, I felt betrayed. I became grumpy and miserable. The best way I can explain it is to say that my sunglasses had thumb prints all over them. The thumbprints were not other people putting their thumbs over my eyes; it was me. I had to learn how to clean my glasses so that I could see.

I remember listening to a lot of music to try to get to a contemplative place. John Michael Talbot, who had once been with the group Mason Proffit but left secular music behind to create beautifully serene, guitar-based Christian music, was my choice. But the lava of self-loathing just kept boiling up. It was the worst of rejections; the worst of failures. I didn't feel suicidal, or that my life was over, but that my destiny was to be in pain. I thought, "Alright, well I'm just fucked for the rest of my life, so I might as well deal."

I didn't deal, though. I would suppress the pain as much as I could, thinking I could just gradually learn to live with it, as if I had lost a limb or something. Somehow I could get to a "new normal," and this pain would just be part of me, like the shape of my hands. But suppressing it didn't work, it just inflated the pain until I was bathing in it.

Eventually, I got bored of being in pain and did something smart; I got a therapist.

Meg told me that I was like an onion, and to get to the heart of what was wrong, I had to peel myself apart, layer by layer. When we started meeting, she asked me, "Why can't you say, this is not good for me? When do you come first?"

Meg's mantra to me, besides always asking myself if a situation was the best thing for me, was, "Chris, live. Put yourself on the list to be reciprocated, because you *deserve* reciprocity. Everyone does."

I asked her, "Why haven't I chosen it?"

"That's why we're here—to figure that out"

Being in therapy was almost like being a child again, but consciously. Meg told me I had to confront the pain I was in, but that I also had to get my mind off of it a little bit.

She asked me, "What's your hobby?" I realized that when I was married, I had suppressed my hobbies and interests, as if I couldn't be the person I had been before. I don't know why I did that. I still did a few things, but not as much as I did before. So I immersed myself in electronics and sound recording again, and computers, and learned everything I could. I studied how to troubleshoot information technology (IT) and sound devices, learned how to design and build, and learned the basics of sound recording.

As I was discovering what I truly loved, I stopped playing music. I realized that I wanted to do was be the power behind the scenes for works of music because that's what gives me the "Wow!" factor. Playing no longer did that for me. Watching someone else play and being able to record it so that their sound comes through in the best way possible gives me more pleasure than playing music myself.

For instance, I love going to watch Damion perform with the Washington D.C. Chorus, because he's the more accomplished musician. My new goal in life is to be a credit in a movie—executive producer, music director, audio engineer, director, or other behind-the-scenes role. That's where I feel most creatively challenged, by working with technology to produce art.

I messed around with digital recording and replication when I wasn't working for the bank. I recorded a lot of live music, ripping and burning them to compact discs and audio files, and playing with them. I would take a song and break it down into multiple tracks, and build it back up again. This was before the mp3 formats shook up the music world. When I worked with sound recording, I felt high, and excited. It's the closest I think I'll ever feel to being a Mom giving birth.

I'd take the live music sessions I had recorded, bought, or found and turned them into digital files. On the Internet, I found a guy who had a copy of the Van Halen concert from February 1, 1984, that was my religious experience. He sent me a copy, and when it arrived in the mail and I listened to it again, I cried like a baby as I experienced the same religious feeling I had when I was there.

Because I was dead, sexually, Meg had to rebuild me a little bit at a time, almost like an automobile transmission. It might sound crazy, but I had to mentally reconnect with my sexual being and resuscitate it. Not only did I have to work out what happened with Helen but I had to get through what I called "the Catholic guilt bullshit" too.

When Meg asked me, "What excites you?" I didn't quite know what to say; I don't think I had ever considered it before. Meg gave me what she called the sexual attraction test. There was a scale from one to ten, and I had to try to fix myself on the scale of what she called my sexual appetite.

For example, she asked, "On a scale of one to ten, with one being Helen and ten being with Pamela Anderson," — this was my scale, and Pamela fit my understanding of a sex machine—"where would you fall on the scale, to be fulfilled sexually by a woman?"

I said, "Probably 9.8, because nothing's perfect."

That's just me being honest, y'all. I love intimacy. I used to make jokes with my female friends who told me that their husbands were not paying any attention to them. I'd say, "Give me your phone. I'm going to make the call and tell your man, 'Do you realize you have a babe for a wife, and you have to treat her right?' "

The ladies loved it.

I worked for the bank for many years, and I liked many of the people I worked with, but some of the executives were so wound up, their assholes could produce diamonds. It was if they were never able to let go, be silly and have fun at work.

When we all got conference call numbers, I wanted to choose seven numbers that could I easily remember, instead of the numbers they had assigned, which I could never recall when I needed to use them. So, I called customer service and asked if I could change my seven-number code to my own personal one. The first thing that came to my mind was Jenny's number. Do you know that song from the '80s?

"Why would you want to do that?" the lady asked. I thought, "Oh my God, get a life! Can't we just make these things easy for once?"

"Please change it to 867-5309," I said.

She replied, "OK, if you want to."

"You never heard of the song?" I was incredulous.

"No," she said flatly.

Well, she didn't get it. So I'm hosting conference calls, and everybody was so serious, following protocol. I would get a standard response when we started meetings, like, "Chris, thanks for hosting the conference call." I would always start off the call by asking, "By the way, did everybody get the trick of what my code was? 867-5309?" Inevitably, of course, someone would say, "Oh! Jenny!" It would loosen everybody up, and we'd be off topic for the first 15 minutes, getting to know one another. To me, it was hilarious, but it was also a way to break the ice, connect with people and quickly find common ground. Then we could get back to work.

My position in the credit card division required continuous travel. When somebody else is paying for your food, and part of your job is rewarding folks with time out of the office— lunches and dinners and after-work drinks—it is very easy to let healthy diet habits slip. Of course, I didn't have any healthy diet habits to begin with!

My typical week was like this: I'd leave on Monday to go to the airport, and I would eat fast food during the day. Dinner would consist of hotel food, which is very rich and flavorful, and then for the rest of the week I'd be eating out. Restaurant and hotel food, five days a week, at high-end places to reward the people I was training—Del Frisco's, Ruth's Chris, Morton's Steakhouse, and on and on, with junk food in between. Maybe the occasional fruit plate. I'd always use broccoli as my out—"I had some broccoli, so I had my vegetables today." Restaurant portions are huge, of course, so I had no portion control.

I never really got into drinking alcohol. I might have one drink if I was out with a team, but I never wanted to be out of control. I know alcohol makes some people loose and apt to say anything, but it makes me sleepy and mopey. Drinking makes me want to hide under the covers. I never liked feeling drunk, either.

Food to me was a comfort that kept on giving. Many times I felt out of control because of timing—you know, timing to get to the airport, on the plane, checked in and to my meetings—and I would feel wound up and tight. Greasy food was almost like a lubricant for me to get relaxed. So my life was just work and eat, work and eat, and my weight went up and up.

On top of that, I wasn't exercising at all, not even taking more than the walks I had to take to get to the next meeting or destination. I recharged with sleep, and usually I would pretty much crash when I got back home. I put so much energy out to be "on," that without naturally replenishing myself with healthy energy, I had to crash and let my body figure it out.

In 1999, I thought I had finally healed from Helen. I thought I was ready for some sexual combustion. Inside, I heard a quiet voice insisting, "Chris, you're the one that's important. What is important is not your job, or who you have." But I blocked that voice out, because it was too painful to think about myself.

I met a woman who worked at one of our banks in Richmond, Virginia, in one of my training classes, and we became really good friends. When I traveled down to Richmond, she became the person that I looked most forward to seeing. We'd hang out at a local bar, play music and pool, and flirt. I began to feel that strange fluttering in my stomach that might be love, but I was hesitant to move things forward. So she made the first pass, which was great, of course, because then I knew I could trust her.

She was at a point in her life when she was on her own and settled into a house after going through a divorce. I would stay at her place in Richmond as much as I could, and we became chemically connected, sexually. Our relationship was a heart-pounding, sweaty experience at first. She was incredibly open and free sexually, and I was intimidated by that, because I never felt that free. I wished, fervently, that I could be. I could give of myself, as before, and she received my attention and reciprocated it. Doesn't that sound great? Well, I didn't know what to do with the reciprocation part.

Things between us were really great for our first year until we hit turbulence. I was getting everything I wanted from the relationship, but I didn't know what to do with it, because I still carried around the deep pain and crushed self-esteem from my first marriage. She began to feel neglected. We got into arguments about whether or not I was being faithful on the road, or looking at other women, which I guess is a common problem, but I couldn't seem to get her to believe in me. I was doing extremely well at the bank, which meant that if we had any kind of disagreement, I had an easy escape: work. I could go to Seattle, Dallas, or even Las Vegas, to visit my call centers.

When we had a chance to turn it around—to break up because we weren't working—I was called back to Charlotte.

I was driving on the 495 Beltway down to Virginia Beach to do a training session with a series of banking centers when I got a call from a senior executive whom I greatly admired. She was one of those mentors in life that you never forget, especially in business. She was a Mom, she was a successful executive, she was funny, she was tough when she needed to be, and she was caring when she needed to be. She called to tell me about an opportunity she had for me.

The position was in marketing, and she said she wanted to bring me down to Charlotte and "stretch me a little bit."

I said, "Great, when's the interview?"

She answered, "This is the interview."

At that point I was sitting in Beltway traffic, not moving much, and my career, my happiness, and my ass were all on the line. I had to choose in a matter of seconds. In this pivotal moment, when I should have asked for more time to consider such a major change in my life, I chose to mount this major obstacle instead of stay where I was and continue in the position that made me so happy.

I was happy in Columbia. I was challenged, I was growing, and I was in touch with my emotions again. But at that moment I felt that if I turned down this opportunity, everything I'd worked for in my life would disappear. I was getting respect from Aunt Phyllis because of the bank job and my success, and Momma Cille was happy, too. I was terrified that I would end up without any family support. It had been a hard road when Aunt Phyllis and Momma Cille had not approved of my relationship, and they were constantly asking me to come home.

I could have said, "I need a day or two to think this over because it's a lot to process." It was the end of August, and I had to be in my new position by October. I told my friend Tony, "I don't want to do this."

He said, "Don't do it, then."

I told him, "I have no choice." I accepted the job for all the wrong reasons—more money, more responsibility, more respect—and went back to the city that I had promised myself I'd never return to again. When I called Momma Cille with the news, she was elated.

"Oh, Chris, I knew you were going to come back home!" she exclaimed. "We're so happy!"

I was miserable. Of course my girlfriend asked, "What am I going to do?" So I asked her to move to Charlotte with me. I remember when I made that suggestion that it didn't feel *right*. If I had taken the chance to be real with her, and with myself, who knows how things would have turned out? I could have taken that opportunity to seize the truth of myself right then. But that's not what happened.

Today, I'm highly over-protective of my decision making. I take my time, and it's my right. If somebody tells me I have to make a decision right now, I'm calling foul. Because if a job or someone needs me that bad, they can get me a day from now while I think things through. But at that crossroad in my life, I feel as if I sold my soul. It was the wrong thing for my girlfriend to come to Charlotte, even though she accepted a different job with the bank, and started working in the real estate business, which was her passion. She gave up everything she had to try it out for me there, and even though it didn't work out, I respect the fact that she took that chance.

I had a terrible go of it during my first year in Charlotte. I was put into a job that I was not qualified for, and if not for my advocates, I would have been fired or laid off. Eventually, my business development and selling skills saved me.

I finally moved to that area of town in which I had always wanted to live. Waxhaw was on the edge of a very well-off neighborhood in south Charlotte, with palatial houses and big lawns. I bought a new house in a new subdivision, and it was enormous—4,000 square feet. I bought a new car, and I was making six figures. Just what I thought I wanted.

My girlfriend had her own issues, too. You know, when two wounded people are trying to be healthy, it's worse when one person's speaking Greek and the other person's speaking Latin. There were some excellent sexual times when I felt so close to her that it scared me. But everything else seemed so hard. Again, I felt that hard was the way my life was supposed to run. We loved each other, though, and I felt I had to take another chance at happiness. I went shopping for a ring.

In 2002, we took a dream trip to see both the Super Bowl and the Pro Bowl. We went to San Diego for the Super Bowl, then to Maui for a couple of days, and then ended up in Honolulu for the Pro Bowl. I asked her to marry me when we were in Maui.

I didn't realize then what I know now. Now, I was aware of the decisions that I was making. I wasn't in a trance or anything; I was being myself, but I was settling for living with nagging fears and worry. In my peripheral vision, I knew that I might have a better life, but I told myself I wanted the one I was making.

She wasn't happy, either, and we ended up in a kind of in limbo for a few years with an engagement that never turned into an actual marriage. I noticed that she had a lot of self-loathing. She liked to go out and have fun, drink, and get silly, which I did not like to do. I was always worried when we went out; always locked and loaded, afraid of what she might do to embarrass me.

On Christmas Eve 2005, I was sitting at home with her, and I told myself I ought to be content. I had the house, the car, and the girl. The Christmas tree was lit, there were at least fifty presents under the tree with shining wrappings, the house was clean and new, and the couch was luxurious and soft. But inside I was *not* happy.

Together, we really tried. We did have fun. We had good times and turbulent times, and we ended up staying together for one more year. But in September 2006, we broke up. She bought a rental property in the same neighborhood we had been living in, and moved out.

At the end of the relationship, I said to her, "I sincerely wish you peace, joy, health and happiness. I want you to experience what you want to have in life." Because she tried so hard with me, and it couldn't work. The bottom line was we were simply incompatible.

Her place was right around the corner from the house I had bought for us to live in, and life had an ugly tinge for a while. She started dating again, and it seemed like she was trying to make me jealous by dating seven or eight guys in succession. But I decided to turn all my engines off. I had to figure myself out. I had to stop making decisions and living my life in patterns that were not good for me. I told myself I couldn't run away anymore. But I did run away—straight back into the arms of work.

Shortly thereafter, my health started declining. In 2001, I had been diagnosed with high blood pressure, but I started having problems controlling it. Dr. Dougherty put me on medicine to regulate it. After we moved into the Waxhaw house, I was diagnosed with high cholesterol, and started taking medicine for that. But my habits did not change. Instead, it was a food fest. My house had been the party house while we were engaged, and we always had an abundance of bad food. I gained weight. And gained, and gained, and gained. Dr. Dougherty told me I needed to drop some pounds. But I thought I was too busy by then, trying to get myself out of the corporate grind and into my own business.

There was upheaval in the banking business. At my bank, I'd worked on many acquisitions as the bank took what they wanted from their acquired companies and spit out what they didn't want, accelerating profit along the way. Eventually my bank merged with another large bank, and I spent a lot of time at the other bank's northeast headquarters working out the details in order to merge my division with them. It was the first major project I worked on where my division was the smaller unit, because the new bank had a larger credit card business.

Off the clock, my new teammates were great, but during office hours, it turned into a plethora of ego and corporate dysfunction. I learned a lot more about the finance industry from them, but I found myself on the minority side about a lot of key decisions.

At any job, you want to be surrounded by people who are in alignment with you, act like you and think like you; not to be a drone, but to make sure you have the same values. In Charlotte, I was assigned to a boss from the new bank who had worked for my bank before. She was a great person off the clock, but as a boss, she could teach me nothing other than driving me to work myself to death. On top of that, my original peers and people that I was responsible for, my line-of-business managers, couldn't stand her. Talk about being caught in the middle! I began to hate going to work.

I wanted to do more with electronics and sound, and I dreamed about owning my own business. I talked with my cousin Tony about it. Tony has always been my sounding board for business ideas and issues. I told him, "Tony, I've got to get out of this."

At one point I was on the road for three or four weeks back to back; I was traveling to locations all over the country—Dallas, Seattle, Vegas, Los Angeles. When I got back from that traveling grind, I came in about ten minutes late for a Monday morning meeting and my boss chewed me out. After she was done giving me her lecture, I closed my portfolio and went into what I call "authentic mode," which is when I get butt-honest and direct.

I told her, "Listen, effective two months from now, I'm leaving this job."

Her eyes got wide. People at work usually saw me as a happy guy who didn't get bothered by things, so when I dropped the gauntlet like that, I guess it was shocking. I knew how to lead, I knew how to motivate, and I had no problem making decisions. I had always accepted my failures as my responsibility, or jumped up when I was praised, but at that moment I knew I did not need that job anymore.

I remember my words vividly. I said, "I do not need this in my life."

I was a senior vice president and my people loved me, but I was willing to give all of that up. The situation was almost parallel to my decision to leave Belmont Abbey. I felt a strong drive to go and do my own thing, and I was passionate about doing it. I love sound, and I have a passion to see that people get the right answers for what they're looking for, not what I want them to have.

I had made some contacts, and closed my first big sale, which was designing a full-house audio system for a professional football player in Charlotte, and I was getting recommendations and offers from other clients wanting similar things done that looked more appealing to me. I had been with the bank for 13 years, and I no longer felt challenged. I had all the accoutrements; the salary, the senior vice presidency, the top-of-the-line car, but none of that gave me the satisfaction that I got from doing my own work.

The remaining two months were hell for me. First of all, I realized I should have just put in a two-week notice like everybody else, but I wanted to finish the job and do it well. Just like The Police after their Synchronicity tour, I wanted to go out on top. But it was a bad situation. I traveled everywhere doing what amounted to grunt work. The traveling was not necessarily a bad thing because the people I worked with were so great, but I called it the "Chris Lynch Says Goodbye" tour. Many people seemed to be simultaneously upset with me for leaving and happy that I was going to be doing what I really wanted to do. There was of course a lot of stress about coming off a regular salary, but in my heart I believed that I could make it work.

My last day was a Friday, and I wanted to go out very quietly. I packed up what was left of my things into a box, and when I was finished at about 4:30, I sat in my empty cube with it and said a little prayer. "God, thank You for this. I don't know what I'm going to be doing, but give me the strength to do whatever I need to do. Thank You for this opportunity." Then I went to the bathroom, and took a dump, as a symbolic act of leaving all the toxic bullshit there. I walked out, got into my car, and drove down the ramp, and ever since that day, I have never looked back and asked myself, "What the hell did I do that for?"

Momma Cille asked me why I was leaving the bank.

"Because I have to," I told her. "Have faith on it, Ma, please."

From that day forward, Ma prayed for my new company. She'd always ask me questions about how it was going, but never to dissuade or discourage me. She was my biggest supporter. Ma didn't have money to give, but she gave prayers, and that was the biggest investment anybody could ever make in me.

My friends and family helped me with my business; specifically, Tony, Don, and Tom. They were my support and conscience. I considered them my Joint Chiefs of Staff, and Tony was really the head of the Cabinet. With Tony, I could put an idea on the table and ask him what he thought, and he would give me an objective, balanced answer. He would never just say to me, "Yes, Chris, this is awesome," so I never had a blank check with him. If he thought it was great, he would tell me, and if he didn't, he would say why or why not. With him, Tom, and Don, I had business support and a sounding board for every project I considered.

In the beginning, the business was consulting for small business development and electronics. I tried to take every talent that I had honed at the bank and leverage it. If someone called about marketing, commercials or design of home theaters, I was their Jack-of-all-trades. I wanted to be the person that customers would feel comfortable coming to, and I wanted to look like I had a thousand people working for me. I developed my own brand, and I put my logo on whatever I could so that when I traveled, I was my company.

I was stopped in the airport by a fellow traveler once because I was wearing a hat with my logo on it that was also branded by an athletics company. A friend of mine who did promotional items got me a deal with the company that allowed me to keep their logo on the hat. The guy who stopped me asked me if I endorsed that company. I explained that I had an alliance agreement, and he asked me how he could get one, too. I told him my company could take care of that, and we exchanged cards. Those kinds of synchronistic interactions gave me hope to keep on doing what I was doing. Eventually the business evolved into being primarily about electronics customization instead of marketing small businesses. My home address became headquarters. Ideas came left and right. I think that being creative at anything makes you even more confident, and you start to have almost a never-ending well of ideas, but money was very slow in coming.

Six months after that, everything I had worked so hard on suddenly fell apart, and I was a diabetic.

8

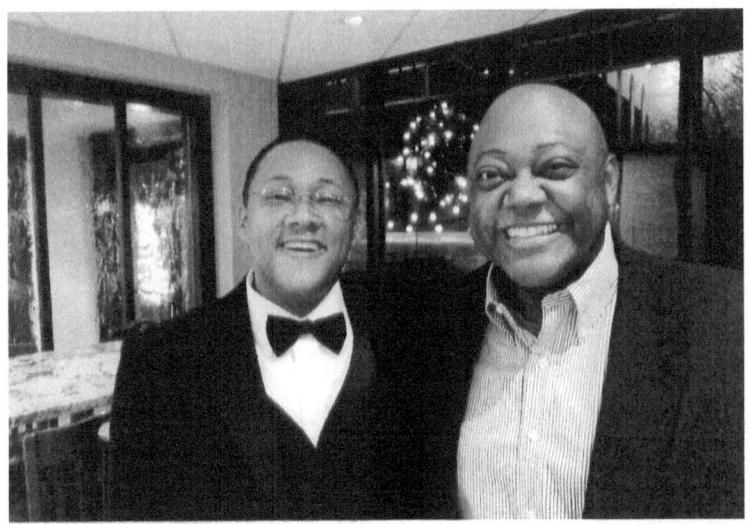

Chris the Diabetic

I was wheeled out of the hospital on Friday.

I remember thinking about everything that I had to do now to stay alive. Just like other mammals, I think humans are instinctively designed to survive, so males especially feel that they have no choice but to be strong. Don's phrase is, "Men, we're the hunter-gatherers." When you're being wheeled out of a hospital in a chair and you're a hunter-gatherer, there's a feeling of helplessness that is intolerable. Some people leave a place like that pissed off at their predicament. I can understand why they might be angry, but I clung to faith. Ultimately, as mere mortals we have nothing. All that we have is God's love, and the rest of it—people, money, medicine, food, shelter, life—is what He gives us through grace.

Fall to me is the most honest and real of seasons. When the hospital door opened and I crossed the threshold to the outside, I took a deep breath. I felt my spiritual inoculation, which gave me permission to take that moment in and feel it. My senses were sharp. I could smell and see things differently.

Then I thought about the bills that were coming, and the fact that I'd been away and didn't know what was going on with my house or my business. I wondered if anybody had been over to check on my home, because I had been very private about what I was going through. I guarded against the vulnerability of intrusion.

When I'm going through something I tend to be very introverted, and when I'm on my own—at mass, or on a plane—I'm not a chatty Cathy. I really try my hardest to harvest those moments because even though I'm an extrovert, I need quiet time to recharge. I'm a boring person when I'm at home. I don't need to go out and party to get my jollies on, or any of that kind of stuff. Yet here was Momma Cille and Blanche fussing over me and getting in my space.

Momma Cille had been over-protective of me growing up, but she became super protective after my time in the hospital because she had almost lost me. There was a comfort in that, because I really needed to be held up now, so I allowed myself to feel her love, but at the same time I wanted to put a little healthy distance between us. Blanche and Momma Cille wanted to immediately come home and stay with me.

We drove around for an hour going in and out of stores trying to find the appropriate insulin. When I went through diabetic training there was a type of insulin that was a little bit easier for me to take because it was in a vial that didn't require refrigeration. I wouldn't have to draw the insulin into a needle; I could just dial a unit back and stick myself with the tiny needle inside it, which is what I wanted to keep doing because I hated needles so much. My prescription when I left the hospital was for 120 units of insulin per day. But we couldn't find the kind I wanted, so I had to get bottles of insulin. We bought a thick package of needles and a sharps container, and then Blanche drove us to my house.

"Ma, I need to go home and I need to be alone," I said. "I need time to process everything." Ma knew and understood me the best, so I think she understood me, but the Lucille Lynch in her was insisting on holding on to me.

"I'm going to make sure you get everything you need," she replied.

"Ma," I insisted, "I just want to go home, take a shower, sit in my quiet little cocoon and just be with this for a minute."

When she dropped me off she said, "Chris are you sure?"

I said, "Ma, it's alright. Just let me go."

For most of my life, when I felt pain, I would stuff it down, put it away, and focus my attention on others. Now, I would never say that helping others is a bad idea. But not focusing on my pain helped put me on a collision course with diabetes. I thought I had acknowledged my fears and was learning how to deal with them. But all I had done was extend the crucible. I had to find a new way to live, and that began by accepting how much help I still had to have.

The leaves were falling when I walked into the house, and I felt weighted. Boy, did I have a lot of shit to do. I sat down; I didn't cry or get mad. I just sat with the disease and became one with it. After a while I became conscious of time. My new reality was being conscious of when to eat, to check my sugar, and when I had to take more insulin.

I didn't have anything in the refrigerator except sugary drinks. I looked at those bottles, and said to myself, "This is poison. This has got to get out of here. I can't look at it anymore." I immediately threw it all away. There was a whole bunch of food that almost killed me in my kitchen pantry, and I threw all that poisonous stuff out. It hit me that I was really lonely, and I wished I had someone significant in my life because I wanted to be held and cared for. But right then, it was just me. So I picked up my own load, and dealt with it. It was to become a character building block.

There was still the problem of no health insurance and no money, so the first person I called was Damion. I said, "Damion, I have nothing, and I have to take this stuff or I will die." Damion said, "Chris, no problem." He acted as my healthcare, because he loaned me the money I needed to go to the doctor and pay for my medicine. You couldn't have asked for more of a saintly action than that.

I was sitting in the bathroom at the vanity where my ex-girlfriend used to do her makeup, looking at a needle, the sharps container, and the insulin. Everything that Ashleigh had trained me to do in the hospital, I had to do now. I was petrified, and hope-filled, and worried, and faithful,

89

and all those emotions were running together inside of me. I had to give myself a shot, because now if I don't take insulin, I'm going to die. There was no IV to back me up, no nurse or Momma Cille to chide me or make jokes with me.

I told Damion, "I'm sitting here with this needle, and I've got to stick myself, and I'm scared."

He said, "Chris, pray. And turn on music." It's funny; music has been an integral part of my life, but I had forgotten about music at that moment. Damion reminded me of my lifeline. In my bathroom, I had the ability to listen to SiriusXM radio, so I turned on The Boneyard, which is a hard rock station. You know—Van Halen, Rush—and suddenly I was back in the zone again. I just started thinking, rock and roll, me and music, the needle and the insulin; I have to do this three times a day.

The temptation was there for me to call Blanche. Momma Cille had said, "Now Chris, if you need to take your medicine, you can call Blanche, and she'll come over there and give you the shot." But I said to myself, "I can't do that, because there will be times where I will not be around Blanche." I said, "I will do this. This is mine now. I have to own it."

I pictured how the nurses did my shots in the hospital as I drew the insulin into the needle. I remembered all the episodes of "Emergency" and "ER" and other medical shows I had watched where nurses gave shots. At the same time, I wanted to have a nervous breakdown! I felt as if I was at the bottom of Mt. Kilimanjaro, Mt. Fuji *and* Mt. Rainier—they were all stacked up on top of each other, and I had to climb up over the summit to get through this disease. I looked at it; I embraced the hills, and I said, "OK, this is it." I pressed the insulin into my thigh.

As soon as I took that first insulin shot on my own, I embraced the fact that I was a diabetic. I took a sticky note and I wrote a motto to put on the mirror as a reminder to take my shots. It said, "Diabetes, you are not welcome in my body." Eventually I had a couple of other phrases; motivational speeches to myself.

I don't think anyone called that night. Most people didn't know what had gone on, because I had lost contact with almost everyone I knew for four days. I think Tom came down, or he called; he had seen that Momma Cille dropped me off. It made me feel really good to know that he was there emotionally.

Tom is a guy that jokes with me, especially about male bonding stuff. He'll say stuff like, "Hold me!" and I'll come back with, "Don't even get near me!" Or I'll flip the bird at him and he'll say, "Yes, folks, we're bonded like brothers!"

I think people were scared by seeing me in that vulnerable of a state. When I saw how my friends and family reacted, I saw how fear and vulnerability connected; I understood how my own fear came from avoidance of that kind of nakedness. I realized I had to climb out of, not only the diabetes hole, but a financial hole as well.

I remember praying, "God, I know now I'm here for a reason, and that you spared me to show me that." I had accepted my own death the night before I went into the hospital; I accepted inevitability. I knew now I had no control over my own life; that control was an illusion because my life belonged to God. God was with me every moment. But I started fighting that reality. I felt like I was out of place because I was in this big house without anyone. I looked around at all my neighbors and friends and relatives, with their kids and wives and husbands—their support networks—and all I had was me. It hurt. What I really should have been doing, which I can do now, was say Thank You.

Getting in the habit of balance, the yin-yang of hypo- and hyperglycemia until I knew completely how to maintain my health, was crazy. At the end of many days, I felt like shit; like an invalid. I didn't have much energy, so I watched TV. I am a news junkie! I love keeping up with what is going on in the world and in the Financial Industry. Fox News and Fox Business are my networks of choice to watch daily! Their shows informed me, entertained me and gave me a connection to the world that I felt not so part of during my time just out of the hospital.

When I had to get my mind off the pain, cartoons and the babes on Fox News got me through: girls, comedy, and of course, music. I remember getting irritable if the women on Fox would wear pants. I'd yell at the TV, "No! I want to see your legs!" Then I'd think. "Clearly I need Valium in addition to insulin because I'm such a mess that I'm yelling at the screen about pants." But I have to tell you, if I was the President of Fox News, I'd make skirts a mandatory thing! That's how I got through the day sometimes.

Tom would come by a lot and hang out with me. We'd laugh and talk and tell each other stupid jokes and bad lines from movies. I had some very bad days. One day I ate three bags of candy—I was trying to give myself a little sugar to balance me out, but I binged and had too much. I guess I was just learning my limits!

When I went to see Dr. Dougherty for the first time after being released from the hospital, our visit began with a lecture. "Well, Chris, you know I told you so!" He didn't really use those words, but he reiterated that there had always been a high probability that I would become diabetic. I had brought my hospital release documents, and Dr. Dougherty let me know that I had been pretty sick.

He asked, "Chris, how are you feeling right now?"

"I feel like I just got off the Love Boat after six months," I answered. I had been taking the 120 units as prescribed, but I was feeling rocky all the time—woozy and sleepy.

"You're probably on too much insulin," he said. "Why don't we take that afternoon shot away from you and replace it with pills?"

"Oh God, thank You!" I was thrilled to lose one of those needle sticks. "How about the other two shots?"

He laughed, but said, "No, Chris. Your numbers are still bad."

Dr. Dougherty put me on MetFormin that day, and my routine changed a bit, so that I was taking shots in the morning and the evening, and MetFormin pills in the middle of the day. Things started to get better, and I slowly stopped feeling like a guest who overstayed his Love Boat "Welcome aboard!"

But it wasn't exactly party time. What I began to call "the needle situation" was bad. It affirmed two things in me, though. One was I will never, ever, *ever* in my life be a drug addict with needles, because I hated taking a shot and sticking myself. I remembered hearing that some guys from one of the metal bands I loved were injecting Jack Daniels in their veins to come down from the coke or whatever drug they did, and I thought, "You idiots! I've got to stick myself with insulin from a pig or a cow to live. Why would you ever do this to yourself when you don't have to?"

The second affirmation was, "I'm coming off insulin, because this is *bullshit*." I got an attitude about it, like Samuel L. Jackson, I said, "Oh, hell no!" I looked at that summit and I started cussing at it. Maybe most people, when they become diabetics, they just lie down and say, "OK, I'm a diabetic." I was the strange dude; I was only going to be a diabetic *temporarily*.

I asked Dr. Dougherty, "What is the chance of me coming off insulin?"

He said, "Chris, that's not even the conversation I want to have with you because you are so in the woods right now."

I insisted. "Doc, give me the numbers."

"For you, one out of a thousand."

I smiled. "I'm the one!"

He shook his head. "Chris, I admire your optimism, but at this point you are too deep in the woods." He knew my family. He knew about the amputations and the sugar packets and the Bayer urine sticks.

Despite the low self-esteem I have battled, I've always believed that when nobody else believes in you, you must believe in yourself. And if you believe in yourself, God believes in you. Knowing God believed in me gave me fuel so that whenever I needed to get anything done I could say, "Jesus and I will do it correctly." So I said, "OK, Jesus, come with me and I'll deal with any obstacle."

My first hurdle was health insurance. When I left corporate America to run my own business out of my house, I couldn't afford it. Everything I had went into my business. Going without healthcare carries a stress load as a diabetic that I can barely describe. I can say that you constantly have to look over your shoulder; you are always thinking of the worst possible scenario and how to avoid it. I couldn't get involved in any situation where I could get hurt. For example, if somebody asked me, "Hey, can you come and help me build something?" I had to say no, or I had to watch how I would put a screw into a hole without getting scratched. I had to take those kinds of things into consideration, because I couldn't just go to a doctor.

The second hurdle was what I called the clusterfuck collision, because every emotion I had ever held back seemed to just come spilling out of me. The physical hurt brought back old emotional hurts, and I had to change the way I reacted to them. I had to start standing up for myself emotionally. I was still smiling, but now I wanted that smile to be authentic.

Lastly, I hadn't started going back to mass yet, even though I had experienced that inoculation of faith with Bishop Curlin. I was still in something of a fog from my illness; I was still healing. I often felt the urge to go to mass; Ma continually pleaded, "Chris, when are you going to mass?" But I would be sitting there thinking, "I don't know how I'm going to pay for the gas to get there." I ended up selling $50,000 in recording gear to try to keep paying my mortgage, but my business was on hold, and eventually I lost my house.

I was dependent on that stupid little needle and it pissed me off. I was mad at myself for getting to that point. I kept saying to myself, "Here I am, just like Aunt Phyllis and my grandfather and all those other people. Fuck this. I'm not going to be that." You know, diabetic ketoacidosis was the same disease that killed the Casey Johnson, heir to the Johnson & Johnson fortune, barely a year and a half after I suffered from it.[5] For some reason I had been spared. God said, "It's not your time yet."

I sat down one day and made a list of things I didn't have: no Mom, no money, no honey, no house. I never got to the point of suicide, but there was a point at which I wanted to die. I wanted to be away from the pain and the loneliness and that pit of self-loathing that I was sinking into. It wasn't a fun place.

When I lay down in bed that night after I had taken my shot, it felt good to be in my own bed, but at the same time ghosts and shadows of the past came back to me. With memories of how I had been before all this happened, and the loneliness, I was a mess. Like a big, mildewy mop, that's how I felt. And I was scared, really scared.

My fear and my faith were colliding, so I was fighting that battle and battling the disease itself. Imagine all of that angst in one person, walking. It's the toughest thing I've ever been through in life. I tie my suffering to the suffering of Christ, even though Christ suffered much harder than I did. Still, pain sucks, and it was time to embrace what Ashleigh, Dr. Kamath, Dr. Dougherty, and all my medical professionals were saying. I told myself, "Now, I own my body. I've got to learn how to keep it healthy." To do that, I had to learn my numbers, and learn how to eat.

---

5 Associated Press, "Casey Johnson Cause of Death: Diabetes Neglect," February 4, 2010.

Dr. Dougherty gave me the numbers I had to aim for. For example, if my blood glucose stayed within a range of 120 - 130 mg/dl before I took my morning shot, it would be a good indication that I needed to lower my insulin intake. The formula for getting healthier, which I still follow, is this: You and your doctor should have the most intimate relationship you can possibly have. Together you have your lab work, your body chemistry and your genes. Your doctor interprets for you what all those things mean and how your body is doing.

You know how some people talk about "being in the moment?" Well, your labs are a record of your body in a moment of time. You and your doctor devise a process of health around those facts. Based on my labs, Dr. Dougherty gave me that blood sugar range to shoot for.

I felt the word "dependence" for the first time. I hated being dependent on insulin, and upon making sure that I'm putting the right food in my body. The dependence made me mad, because I was so afraid. The first thing I did was, I stopped eating anything that contained sugar. It seemed obvious to never eat sugar. But that led me to having several hypoglycemic episodes because I became sugar-deprived.

I first reached out to my cousin Patrick. Even though Damion and I are brothers, I talk more to Patrick because we have so much in common. We love sports and we're both salespeople, so I felt very comfortable being vulnerable with him. He made it fun and easy for me to learn how to eat better.

When my friends and family learned about my diabetes, they gave me a lot of advice, and it was spinning me in circles. For example, there was the packet controversy. Some people said, don't eat the yellow packets because yellow packets have a sweetener that is bad for you. Others said, don't eat the blue packets because blue packets have a chemical in them that can hurt you. It was, yellow is this, blue is this, pink is this. It was too many thises!

Patrick gave me tactical and practical help. He told me what to do, and gave me exercises to do. He made eating better a challenge; like a little adventure. I didn't even know how to shop for the right food, so I was afraid to go to the grocery store, and I was terrified about having to start cooking for myself. It was as if I had to learn how to be an adult all over again. Thinking about doing it by myself made me feel like I wanted to just collapse. I thought of what Harry Truman said when he took the presidency over from Franklin Roosevelt. It was something like, "I don't know if you ever had a bale of hay fall on you, but that's what I feel like right now."

For example, Patrick would tell me, "Chris, go to the grocery store and find this item and this item." He made learning how to eat better like a scavenger hunt.

Patrick asked me, "What do you eat? How do you go to the grocery store?" Once I realized what I liked to eat, Patrick helped me change those things so I could eat safely. He helped me take what I had learned in the hospital and at the doctor's, and turn it into practical habits for eating and shopping and exercising. And my habits changed tremendously.

I was like a drug addict weaning off drugs. Fatty foods were my drugs. I think it's probably easier to come off cocaine than fatty foods, because frankly, they taste so good. I was addicted to my comfort foods and sugary drinks. Every decision that I made going to the grocery store was about getting rid of old habits and starting new ones. I became a sponge. I was learning a lot about nutrition, how to refuel my body, and how to get my body chemistry back. The first 60 days really sucked. They were filled with a lot of learning, a lot of fear, a lot of agony, and a lot of questions. Patrick was very patient with me. I would call and ask him about anything I didn't understand on a food label, and he was always helpful. His joke to me was, "At least you're going to be one less death statistic."

Once I got into a groove and started physically feeling the good that was coming about as a result of what I learned, it became even more fun to go out and learn about new foods and how to cook them. Patrick said it's better if you can replace a carbohydrate with a vegetable. So instead of having more carbs to feel full, I would double up on low-fat meat and have more vegetables. For example, I would get chicken and season it with low-sodium everything. Then I'd cook it using virgin olive oil with red and green peppers, and onions. I'd stir that together with Worcestershire sauce and eat it, and it made me feel healthy.

I started thinking, "More vegetables!" The greener the vegetable, the fresher the vegetable, the better. I lean towards broccoli, but I also love turnip greens. I would make things like turnip greens and pico de gallo and the peppers and onion medley. When you start doing that, it becomes a good habit. Then I realized if I could do this to chicken, I could do it to pork, and if I could do it to pork, I could do it to beef. I would try some things, and not everything was successful! I also started learning what to stay away from, which for my severe situation is pastas and rice.

By the 60th day or so, after Thanksgiving, it all started getting easier. Now I tell people if you really want to be on the right diet, eat a diabetic diet, because a diabetic diet is a way of life, not a trend. For me, everything had to change: breakfast, lunch, dinner, snacks; what I ate, what I didn't eat, how I ate it, when I ate it, why I ate it. For instance, now that I've changed, I've fallen back in love with vegetables, and when I don't have enough of them, I miss them. I used to drink sugared soda like it was water. Sometimes I would drink four sodas in a day. Eventually I found a great substitute, a flavored water that tastes like soda but doesn't have much in it other than all-natural flavoring, and it's delicious. After that, I basically said to people who wanted to give me advice, "Thank you for your prayers, but you don't need to pray for me. Pray for yourself that you don't get as bad as I got. Know that I'm in good hands with my doctor."

I started getting into a groove that I felt a bit better about. I could start to try to deal with my business and finances. At the same time, I felt like laying down and being sad all the time. I felt a tenseness. That's the best way I can describe it. Inside I was this scared, intimidated, fear-filled and sick Chris. I still had a long road ahead of me. But gradually my health got better.

Dr. Dougherty started dropping my insulin requirements as my body started to heal. So I went from 120 to 100, 100 to 90, 90 to 80, 80 to 75 units; see how it all works? On February 5, 2009, I stopped taking insulin shots altogether. I'm still on blood pressure and cholesterol medication, but my blood glucose level averages about 117 per day. To go from a level of 1469 mg/dl and taking 120 insulin units per day to 117 mg/dl, and no insulin? That's God.

9

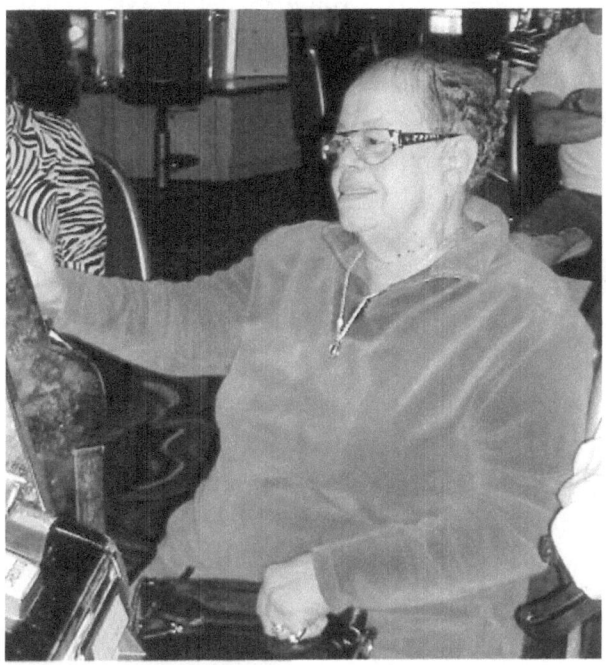

Believing and Receiving

Aunt Phyllis died in the little hospital room that we
made up for her at home, and Ma was declining, too.

We used to call it the breakfast room. I felt so sad for her because she was
lying in her bed, dying. But she had this very peaceful aura about her.

I remember that I rushed around the house and grabbed everything I
could find that was Catholic—holy water, rosaries, scapulars—and made
this little shrine around her bed. She and I shared a joke when she moved

into that room. Barack Obama was running for President, and when I was visiting Damion up in D.C. one time, I brought back two political buttons to Charlotte. One was for Hilary Clinton and one was for Obama. The Obama one was for Aunt Phyllis and the Hilary one was for Momma Cille.

I told Aunt Phyllis, "I want you to go out in style, so just in case you go, I want you to know that I put your Hilary button on your blouse." She'd protest. "No, get that off me!" Then I'd show her the Obama button instead. She was not a fan of Mrs. Clinton! When she was able to give me her last "audible," which was what I called her giving me specific instructions, she said, "Chris, please make sure that your business is good and that you do a good job with it."

I remember I held her hand, and the anger that I wanted to feel for all the times she punished me and made me feel bad about myself did not arise. I pushed whatever was left of it aside and allowed myself to feel her peace. I believe that was a moment from God where I felt healing between Aunt Phyllis and me. I was able to let all that go, and leaned over her.

"Aunt Phyllis," I told her, "Thank you for everything. I forgive you. Please forgive me. God bless you, and I love you."

She couldn't answer me because she was having such a hard time breathing, but the look in her eyes told me she forgave me, too. She died a few hours later of congestive heart failure and complications from diabetes.

While I was working on stepping down from insulin, I spent a lot of time visiting with Momma Cille. I couldn't seem to find a job, but I was getting by living off of the proceeds from the sale of my recording equipment. Money was a constant worry.

I did some research for Ma about Saint Mungo, her family's namesake and patron saint. Born with the name Kentigern in Scotland, it is said that his teacher called him Mungo, which means "dear one" in the Welsh language. He became the Roman Catholic Bishop of Strathclyde, in Glasgow, Scotland, and died early in the 600s. One of the miracles attributed to him was the resurrection of his teacher's pet bird.

Momma Cille's maiden name was Mungo. I collated the research I found and brought it to her, and her reaction was typical. She acted as if I had brought her a million dollars in cash.

"Oh Chris," she said, "Let's look at this!" She was so proud, and it was a beautiful thing. We talked about getting a group together with Bishop Curlin to visit his church and shrine. She wanted to kneel at St. Mungo's tomb and pray. We were never able to do that, but I gave her a little glimpse of the place by bringing her the clippings and web articles. I could tell that she just relished that moment we had together, and when I saw her after that she told me she had been "reading that book you brought me." She called everything a book—magazines or any sheaf of paper.

Christmas time came quickly after I got out of the hospital, and Ma told me she wanted a GPS device. She admired the one that I had in the car I managed to hold onto for a little while. Later on that car was repossessed. She said she wanted the GPS to travel, but she kept calling the device a "GSP."

I asked her, "Ma, where would you and Blanche go with a GPS?"

"Oh, we'd go to Cherokee! We could plot the course on the GSP, and Blanche and I could go to all of our favorite places, like BJ's Warehouse."

She was utterly sincere, which was hilarious! I considered getting her one, just to hear her say to me, "Now Chris, where can we go now?"

One of Momma Cille's favorite places was Las Vegas, NV because she could gamble. We had often taken family trips there, and that spring we all went out to Vegas again. To this day, I wish that I had taken some kind of recording device with me, because some of her best lines came out of that trip.

Momma Cille was excellent at picking out what she called "flimflammers," or people who would try to screw you over by presenting deals that were too good to be true. That said, she fell for the biggest racket of them all, because Momma Cille was a big believer in. . . slot machines.

In Vegas, we stayed at the Rio, and I would walk around with her in the hotel and casino. She got around with the help of a walker that I christened her Escalade, and it was slow going, but I didn't mind because I loved hanging out with her. So we're walking and stopping every little bit to rest, and she's saying hello to everyone that passes as if we were at church.

We were actually in Vegas during Holy Week, the week before Easter, which was funny in and of itself. The Rio at that time featured the Chippendale dancers, and as we were walking, some of the cocktail waitresses walked past us. Momma Cille could not believe all the flesh they showed.

"Chris," she exclaimed, "Why don't they have any clothes on?"

I died laughing. I said, "Ma, it's Vegas, the skimpier the better!"

"But it's Good Friday!" she said.

She asked me who they were and what they did, and after I'd told her, she said, "Oh, there must be some frisky stuff going on in there!"

"And you'd probably be right." I shook my head, laughing.

Ma was right-handed, so when she played the slots she would hold what I called her Catholic rig in her left hand. Her Catholic rig was her brown scapular, a Miraculous Medal and her rosary. She would hold that in her left hand and talk to the machine. "Come on, St. Mungo, I'm related to you! Let's make this work!"

She'd make the sign of the Cross, and she said you had to trick the machine by tapping the button instead of pulling the lever. When she'd win, she'd tell me to give her some of her winnings back so she could play some more. When I protested, she would tell me, "Chris now, I'm an old lady. When I'm in heaven I'll be giving y'all the lottery numbers, so I have to at least take my fortune now when I can." She was priceless.

She kept saying to me, "Chris, live your life." Live your life, be good, go to church, love God, love your neighbor, and don't take any mess off anybody. I believe she always admired my strength, but at the same time, she saw a lot of my weaknesses. I know that frustrated her because she wanted to see me succeed, and I wanted to prove my success to her. One of the expressions she used to say a lot was, "I'm going to stay right here." I hear her so many times now saying that to me. One day recently I was out walking around D.C. in the winter air, and I heard her tell me, "Chris, you've got to cover your head. Now, I don't like it that you don't have hair, but you've got to cover that head up, it's too cold out here! I'm not going out, though; it's too cold. I'm going to stay right here."

At mass I often marveled at the way Momma Cille used to take the Host during Holy Communion. I could see that she was taking the Host not only for herself but for all those that she couldn't help. She'd pray with her eyes squinted shut hard. When I pray now, I often say those squinting prayers, where I'm praying desperately that other people are able to experience what I have felt spiritually.

Ma left us on April 17, 2009. She started having heart problems and was admitted to CMC Main in uptown Charlotte, where I was born. She went very fast, and I was present in her room when she died. I had been simply terrified to face Ma leaving me.

I had not gone to mass or to Benediction for a long time. I began to feel the ever-present urge to go, though, and I think God was nudging me because the compulsion to go was always there. Ma would frequently ask me when I was going, and I would think about not even having the money to pay for gas to get there. Things were getting tighter and tighter, and the day was coming when I would hold my last dollar in my hand.

Being with Ma during her last moments was the greatest gift of my entire life. She could not impart any more knowledge to me, which is why I think her passing was so quick. It seemed as if she had just gotten to the hospital, and then she was gone. After Bishop Curlin came in and gave her the Anointing of the Sick, the doctor told us that the next 24 hours were going to tell us how it would go. I felt that it was time to say my goodbyes.

Ma had an oxygen mask on. I stood next to her bedside and said, "Ma, I just wanted to say I love you, and thank you for everything,"

She said, "It was my pleasure. You were always a good child, and I love you too."

She had a washcloth on her forehead that a nurse had placed there to cool her face, but it was making her hair a mess.

She said, "Chris, can you take this washrag off? I don't want to die with this on my head."

As she lay there, I saw a person who I knew from my earliest memories to her last breaths as consistent in her actions. She was a model of unconditional love and a true child of God. I sat there in the room while people came in and out to say goodbye. She died the next day, a Friday, at 1:09 in the afternoon,

When Momma Cille took her last breath, I felt a baton was handed to me. God gave me the grace and peace to witness her leaving me, and it was totally peaceful. She took a final breath, and it slowly drained out. The room was utterly silent and I felt a presence filling the room, and then departing. As I realized she was leaving, I humbled myself before Christ, and all I can tell you is, I understood it. I saw and felt her go, and it was not to death.

There was a very simple cross, on a black string, and a brown scapular that I purchased at the Basilica when I couldn't afford much. I would wear it to mass or whenever I visited the Basilica. I wanted to thank Momma Cille by giving her the two symbols of my faith to take with her. So I had a private conversation with the funeral director and asked him to place my cross and scapular with Ma, under her dress where she would have worn it.

As soon as we buried Momma Cille's body at Belmont Abbey cemetery that following Sunday, I started going back to mass. About three months later, I had a dream. I had forgotten to set my alarm clock, but in my dream I heard three voices waking me up at my normal time. The voices that I heard were Momma Cille, Aunt Phyllis, and a voice that I believe was my Mom, Patricia.

They said, "Chris, get up!"

I shot up in bed, fully awake, and smiled. I felt a graceful peace. Since then, Ma has come to me several times. Since her death, I've been carrying that faith, executing it, living it, being it. Now I have permission to harvest everything that she taught.

I made peace with Ma's "no cross, no crown" mantra. Despite the intense pain and aloneness I sometimes felt, and the awkwardness of being isolated under her protection, I wouldn't trade being her grandson for the world because she made me who I am today. I try to honor her and her memory by my faith, by praying for others, and by my devotion to Mary.

Tony said something to me right after Momma Cille died. He said, "Chris, you know, Momma Cille used to talk about wanting to win the lottery, but she died a wealthy woman."

His words felt like a bucket of cold water being dumped on me, and they shook me hard. It was a revelation of the truth of her. I remember I said, "Zing!" That was the beauty of her life.

Momma Cille showed love throughout everything in my life; the trials, the traumas, the ups, the downs, the people that I dated that she didn't like. When she died, all I could think about was the love that she gave me the best way she could. God took her because she was done.

Several people pulled me aside afterwards to tell me that Ma had a very special love for me. They said she'd talk about me when I wasn't around, saying that she respected me for being tough and vibrant in life. So what I did was accept the truth of it, saying, "Let me embrace what was done, and let me go live my life without fear."

I became hope-filled and blessed with love for myself, because Momma Cille was a walker; she demonstrated her faith and love every day. Now my devotions are an intrinsic part of me; I *want* to go to mass now because I need it, not because it is my duty.

Later that year after Ma died, I went down to visit my buddy Doug in Florida, and attend his wedding. As I was driving down from Charlotte, I felt a quick, quiet, whispering command, and the command was, "It is finished." It continued to resonate in my head the whole time I was in Florida and when I was coming back, and with it came a longing to go back to the DC area.

I called Don first. I guess Don is the person who I usually call to sort of get permission for what I'm contemplating. He's like my gut check.

I told him, "Don, I have to leave. I'm going back to Washington."

I didn't know how I was going to do it. I was getting foreclosure notices because I could not afford my house, but it didn't feel like home anymore. When they turned the dirt in Momma Cille's grave was when I should have said, "I'm outta here!" But it wasn't. I guess I had to catch up to the freedom that was inside of me to go live my life as Momma Cille had said. As soon as I got off the phone with Don, I called Damion and told him I was coming home.

Damion replied, "Chris, I knew you were going to say this, I was just waiting on you to say when."

"Really?" I was surprised.

He said, "Yes, I was having this conversation with my friend Robert, and I told him, 'I'll bet you that Chris is going to come back up here.'"

From October to Thanksgiving, I made preparations. I dismantled my home and cleaned up the clutter of my life. The day I left Charlotte was one of the happiest times I could remember having in a long time. When I pulled away from that house, I could honestly say I tried my best. I gave it my all, and even though I was immersed in failure, I felt like I was doing the right thing.

It was crazy because everything fell into place. I was almost flat broke, but I found a one-way plane ticket for only 36 dollars to Reagan Airport. I moved in with Damion. It took me quite a few months to find a job, but I eventually ended up back in sales—selling audio and electronic equipment for a major company. I lived with friends for a while; it took me about a year to have enough in my budget to afford my own apartment.

In D.C. I learned how to take resources and make them stretch, and I learned to get over some of my ideas which were just, well—bullshit. Like thinking I can't shop at the dollar store, when there's nothing wrong with the dollar store. My masculinity, my humanity, my sanity and my health all collided and when they did, I shook loose a lot of the stupid baggage I was carrying. When you're stripped down to survival—when you just want to be able to buy toilet paper—there's a humility that comes from that.

I remember several times when I was looking for a job, Damion said, "Chris, I'll drive you down to the Metro if you want." But I'd say, "No Damion, I've got to walk." I still have the one pair of shoes I had then as a reminder of that time. I couldn't afford to buy new shoes, so I wore the ones that I had to the bone. I remember walking and realizing that all I had was my own power to get me through. It would be bitter cold in the winter walking back from mass, but I learned to thank God for the little things I had once taken for granted. I would see cars whizzing by as I walked and would pray, "Thank you for my two cars—my right foot and my left foot."

The humility I learned from that is such that I will never go back to what I was before. I used to go to Las Vegas regularly on somebody else's dime, but I don't miss any of that. I don't want to acquire eight houses or six Bentleys, or any of the ridiculous trappings that come from working for those things. When we have no possessions or even hope, there is still something left, and all we have to do is reach for it and believe in it. That's what I did.

My mantra, now, has become this: Believe. Receive. Reciprocate.

How do you believe? Faith requires a stripping down: of your ego, of your petty desires, of grasping for things. When you have let go of everything, you become like a child again. Remember when you were small and you became ill, and the whole world was your sickness—your stuffy head, your sore throat, your headache? Nothing else existed. There was no past, no future. You were just in pain, and you cried out for help so the pain would cease. That is the closest I can come to explaining my belief in God: how a child worships. It stems from my fundamental vulnerability, not from skepticism, arrogance or heady articulation.

It's as simple as saying, listen to the sound of wind or the words of a psalm, and feel the beauty within it. Look intently at the smile of a person talking to you. Receive a hug that someone gives you, and recognize that there's healing in that. When I was in the hospital, the care of the nurses and their touch was a crucial factor in my healing. They helped equip me to deal with the desert of those times. Even unto today.

That doesn't mean I'm flawless or sinless. What it means is that I have experienced the pure love of God. He allowed me to live and have the privilege of talking to you right now. So many times, I have wondered why I was spared. Why did I survive when I should have died? There is no answer available in human knowledge, and I can't even be sure that if God has a reason for it. What I do know is that there's a responsibility that comes with the gift of my life, and it keeps me in check. God heard me over all the years that I was in agony, because the greatness of God was, and is, as close to me as my own breath.

I am more contemplative in my Catholic faith and prayer now. At the Basilica, I can get lost in the mystery of God and see how the arrogance and struggle of all our lives is as nothing before that. When I kneel in front of the Blessed Sacrament and I pray, I am not praying to the monstrance, but to the true essence of love that has given me another chance to live my life the way it should be lived, in peace, joy and happiness. Now I want to invite others into this day.

10

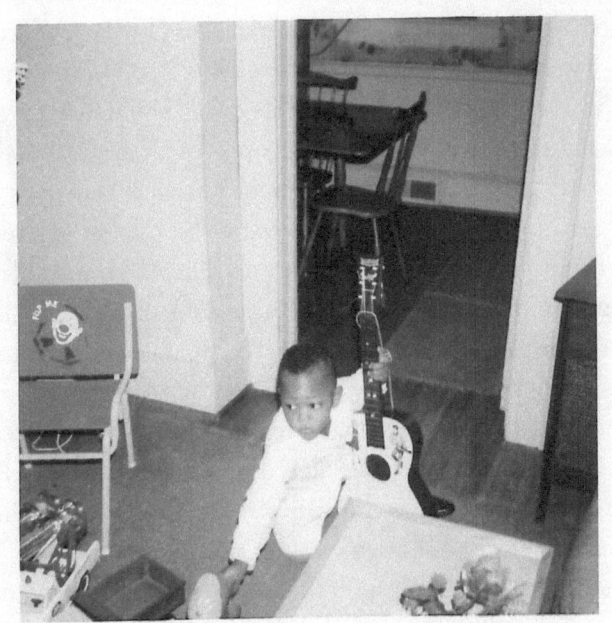

Reciprocate within your reach

Today I no longer take insulin, and people often ask me, "How did you do it?

The magic answer is, say yes and embrace. That's the answer. I know it sounds too simple, but that's what it is. I got over insulin-dependent diabetes because I said, "I can't do this, God. Help me." And it was as if He said, "Go through this, and I'll send you the people and the help you need." His love is right in front of us, within our reach. Everything that you need is right in front of you.

My life wasn't instantly healed; in fact, it was a constant battle of climbing out of a musty hole, making a little progress, and falling backwards. I had lost everything, even my health, but I slowly came back to life. I received everything I needed.

I said before that in my relationships, I had a hard time receiving love from others. I know now that this stemmed from my lack of faith. If God created us, He will take care of us, and we must receive Him with a loving and open heart. When others showed me love, I should have embraced it, gave thanks, and done everything in my power to reciprocate that gift.

Today, I do not have that huge house or that luxurious car, but I feel wealthier now than I ever did. I enjoy the harvest of everyday life. Whether or not you have diabetes, another illness, or are suffering some other trauma, to me there is a simple formula for surviving it all, and that is embracing the fullness of your reality, which at its core is your complete vulnerability as a human being.

I am not here to advance a diet or regimen for diabetics, because every diabetic is different, and every person is different. What I can tell you from my experience is, work with your medical team. Be completely honest with them about everything—how it's going, what you are doing, when you slipped, and how you feel. Without that data, they cannot formulate a plan to help you. They will tell you the numbers you must shoot for, and how to keep those numbers in balance.

You must also embrace your pain. Life is not a continuous series of disasters, but it can seem that way when you try to hold back the reality of the pain in your life. Being alone hurts. Being sick hurts. Being poor hurts. Trying to take drugs or alcohol or bad food will only mask the pain, not relieve it. If you don't accept your pain, you will never be a complete human being, because pain is part of the world which God has given us.

I've had people say to me, "Chris, how can you continue to smile?" Well, my smile now is earned, because I embraced the bottoming out of my life. Saying that does not mean taking on the mantle of your ego by being proud of surviving your trials.

If anyone tries to dissect me, my faith or my experience, they are going to lose because I'm still a work in progress. But I say this to skeptics: if you don't believe, close this book. If you don't have a glimpse of belief in yourself, this will sound like Barney the purple dinosaur on marijuana.

But if you hear what I've gone through, maybe my pain and suffering can help you identify that it's okay to be broken. It's okay to lose a 4,000 sq. ft. house and still have your self-esteem.

My job is to put myself out there and give you this invitation to be loved and cared for. Now, I choose good health. Now, I choose happiness. Now, I choose joy. You don't have to waste any more time: just receive His love and mercy. Believe it and receive it.

Receiving it means you don't have to go look for it, because it is part of the gift of your life. Reciprocating those gifts to others is the natural response to believing and receiving. So instead of looking for love, I'm going to be loving. I'm going to give love, and I'm going to show love—and if I look stupid, so be it. Because when I put my head on my pillow at night, I know who I am. Whereas before, when I played the game of "look at me," I was miserable. I had to live in the right house, in the right neighborhood, make the right money, and on and on. When you reciprocate, the cycle will begin anew.

Today I can say to you that I have peace of mind and I know that I am doing my part. I said, no more to being unhealthy, and God sent me Damion. He sent me Don. He sent me Tony, and Tom, and Deirdre, and Patrick, and Michelle, who helped me to write this book. He sent me laughter. He sent me simplicity. He sent me pain. Now, I'm still struggling every day to be the person I want to be, but I'm aware, and because I'm aware, I want to live by example.

What I look for now is not monastic austerity, but for things that are not going to distort me or distract me away from life. I listen to the voice of God inside of me that says, "Chris, just keep walking, I've got you."

The decision is not for someone else to make for you. The decision is in you. What I encourage you to do is have a discussion with the people that you call your support network and discover what your path is, then walk it. Believe, receive and go reciprocate to others *within your reach*. If your reach is five people, talk to five people. If your reach is a million, talk to the million, but help whoever is within your reach.

The nurses and doctors in the hospital, they helped me in the moment; I was in their reach. It may have been their job, but at the end of the day, it's about human being helping human being. This doesn't mean that you've got to make 50 million dollars to start a foundation, nor that you've got to die penniless. Of course you can do things that empower others, but remember that there is wealth in the shortest prayer. There's wealth in self-esteem. There's wealth in taking a minute and saying to someone, "You are beautiful. You are good. You are kind."

During my diabetic journey, my ultimate receiving moment was when Bishop Curlin said to me, "Chris, my stuff works." I received that guarantee. I said, "God, I receive Your grace." And when I gave to others with a joyful heart, all of those things began to formulate into help for me. Then I felt peace, love and joy again.

After Ma was buried, Don and I went to mass at Our Lady of Bishop Curlin's house. Bishop Curlin told me that Ma had passed the baton of love to me. He told me, "Chris, you are glowing with the strength of the light of Christ." That humbled me. Bishop Curlin had been Mother Teresa's spiritual advisor for years, and knew her intimately. It humbled me that a man who had known her, a woman who was completely filled with Christ and recognized by our Church as a saint, saw that in me.

Now every day I kneel down and pray, "Lord, please use me today. Help me to do what You want, and let it be Your will."

I beg you to do the same, and then watch what will happen in your life and in those around you.

Help Within Your Reach

I am a Roman Catholic, but I could never tell anyone what doctrine to follow, including Christianity. I can only share my experiences, which include my Christian, Roman Catholic faith. My faith practice includes going to weekly mass, and Benediction with the Blessed Sacrament.

I have included Catholic prayers in this chapter that have been of special importance to me, and some web links that you may wish to visit to learn more.

Prayer to Our Guardian Angel

Angel of God, my guardian dear,
to whom his love commits me here,
ever this day be at my side,
to watch, to lead, to guard, to guide.

Prayer of Benediction with the Blessed Sacrament

Lord our God, in this great sacrament
we come into the presence of Jesus Christ,
your Son born of the Virgin Mary
and crucified for our salvation.
May we who declare our faith in this fountain of love and mercy
drink from it the water of everlasting life.
We ask this through Christ our Lord.
Amen.

Web Resources

- For more information about living with diabetes, visit the American Diabetes Association at diabetes.org
- For resources from the Roman Catholic Church, including prayers, liturgical calendars, and other information, visit catholic.org

Acknowledgements

I would like to acknowledge Drs. Kishan and Kamath, and all of the nurses and staff of Carolinas Medical Center-Pineville for their care of me when I suffered from diabetic ketoacidosis, especially Ashleigh Thore, my nutritionist, who was the first to introduce me to my new way of life. Thank you all for bringing me back to an incredible second chance at life. Also, Richard A. Dougherty, MD, and his assistants Tracy, Lori, and Mary, who helped me every step of the way in my journey from 1469 to 120.

To the mighty Van Halen, whose incredible music pumped me up when I celebrated milestones, and kept me up when I felt tired and weak: your music gave me that extra kick in the ass to never stop rockin'!

I will be eternally grateful to my family and friends: Mary Richardson and Blanche Jackson, for helping me to get to the hospital on that fateful day in October 2008; my brother Damion, who was my "healthcare provider" when I could not afford medicine or food; my cousin Patrick, who taught me how to shop and change the way I eat; Tony Silva, my coach, motivation and conscience; Don Russell, my best friend through this entire journey; Tom Richardson, my sense of humor; Reverend William G.

Curlin, Bishop Emeritus of the Roman Catholic Diocese of Charlotte, NC, whose stuff worked and set the tone for my new faith journey; Michelle Tackabery, my dear friend and partner on this project, for pulling this story out of me to tell the world; and finally, my guardian angel, Lucille Mungo Lynch. If it were not for her loving motherly concern pushing me to get to the hospital, I would not be alive today to share this story with you. I hope I made you proud, Momma Cille. May you rest in peace.

Michelle Tackabery would like to acknowledge my husband, Richard Tackabery, for his undying support for this and all my writing projects; Christine Allen, my sister, for her love and confidence in me; and the members of my writing group in Raleigh, North Carolina: Julia Fountain, Judith Valerie, Laurina Uribe, Tina Golian, Jerri Harrell, and Karen Brisendine, who heard pieces of this manuscript and gave critical commentary, advice and feedback during its completion. Finally, I must acknowledge the contributions of Suzanne Hayes Rose, our editor, for her assistance in making this the best book I could write. This is a big hug of thanks for her wisdom and support.

THE END